Opening

the *Cage* of *Pain*

with *EFT*

Also By Rue Hass:

This is Where I Stand:
the Power and Gift of Being Sensitive

The 8 Master Keys to Healing What Hurts

The Discovery Book:
Workbook for EFT and the 8 Master Keys

Opening
the Cage of Pain
with EFT

Let Your Spirit Fly Free

Rue Anne Hass, M.A.

Opening the Cage of Pain with EFT:

Let Your Spirit Fly Free

Edited by Jeremy Berg

Cut Paper Collage Cover Art by Willow Harth

Published by:
Starseed Publications
2204 E Grand Ave.
Everett, WA 98201

ISBN: 978-0-9791700-1-0

Hass, Rue Anne
Opening the Cage of Pain with EFT/
Rue Anne Hass

First Edition: January 2008

Printed in the United States of America

9 8 7 6 5 4 3 2 1 0

Index

Dedication

To everyone everywhere who embraces new ideas with courage, delight, curiosity and creativity.

Acknowledgements

Timothy - for always, all ways, holding a space open for what is possible in me

My mother - who opened a portal into the world for me to enter, and who deserved way more acknowledgment than she ever allowed herself to receive, especially from herself

David Spangler - for his deep wisdom about the sacred in incarnation that points to the living Presence in the phrase "Stand Up for Yourself"

Gary Craig, developer of EFT - for his generosity of spirit and investment on behalf of healing the heart of the world

Chapter 1:

Introduction

Chronic Pain

is

an emotional freedom technique.

This is true of all chronic conditions.

I believe that chronic pain can emerge from years of hiding, holding back, caging, or repressing our deepest self-expression. Chronic pain is the body's expression of emotional and spiritual pain. Pain gets our attention! It is calling us to free our deep spirit.

We are only just learning how to respond to that call, and EFT is our key to the cage. This material on calming and clearing chronic pain will describe some of the primary emotions and beliefs that hold the cage in place, and how we can use EFT to, literally, free our souls.

Overview

This approach to chronic pain emerges from my experience in working with people who have had it. I do not have chronic pain myself, although I have learned that I have the temperament for it. If I had had an abusive family experience instead of "just" the emotionally neglectful one that I did have, I would have been a good candidate for fibromyalgia, rheumatoid arthritis, chronic fatigue, irritable bowel or one of the auto-immune disorders that are baffling medical science.

I have learned from several sources: from wide and deep personal study, from teaching a class for several years with a physician who healed herself from chronic pain, and from working with many, many experts—the people who have the condition themselves. My physician colleague, Nancy Selfridge, taught the class participants (and me) about the enlightened medical approach to fibromyalgia, and I taught them (and her) how to do EFT with fibromyalgia, as well as a different way to think about being ill. Nancy is now Chief of the Integrative Medicine clinic of a Wisconsin HMO. Her highly readable and valuable book, written before our work together, is *Freedom from Fibromyalgia*.

Even though I have become well self-educated in the field of these new disorders, and in the effectiveness of EFT as a treatment modality for them, what I say here are my views only, unless I am quoting someone.

The large frame I want to put around this information is that, in my mind, chronic conditions are not "diseases", so much as they are **the evidence of a spiritual dis-order**. I believe that when the human spirit is confined over time by negative emotions, thoughts, beliefs, or environments, and is not allowed or encouraged to give itself full expression, the resulting anger and grief eventually show up in the body as pain. By "spirit," I mean what is best in us. I believe deeply in our innate goodness. In reading these words, please feel free to substitute your own spirituality for mine. I think it all draws from the same well.

Chronic pain gets our attention. To me, chronic emotional or physical pain is the spirit screaming. The message of the scream is basically "Let me out of here!" Skillful, thoughtful EFT, practiced individually or co-creatively with a practitioner, invites and makes possible the freedom of the human spirit from its cage of negative thoughts and beliefs. We have in our hands a tool that can change everything!

Chronic pain is a technique of the body-mind-spirit that calls us to emotional freedom.

This information will be for *you*, if you have pain or other chronic conditions, and for *you*, if you are a practitioner who wants insight into how to work with it, or both. This is not a definitive treatment of pain disorders. My intention here is to share the beliefs and emotions that create the structure of chronic pain, emotional and physical, and hold it in place. Once we can grasp the structure, we can use our own intuition and the excellent tool of EFT to re-frame and re-build it.

I will begin with a definition of chronic pain from an "enlightened medical perspective," from the energy psychology perspective, and from a spiritual perspective, as I understand it.

An Enlightened Medical Perspective on Chronic Pain

Let's begin with a few words from **Dr. Nancy Selfridge** herself. This is the outline form of her part of the presentation we gave together a few times at the ACEP (Association for Comprehensive Energy Psychology) conference. Here she is talking about fibromyalgia specifically, but most of what she says is true more broadly for chronic pain as well. It will give you an overview.

4

I. A Mind-Body Model for Understanding Fibromyalgia

   1. Is fibromyalgia all in my head?

   • Pain is a complex neuro-physiological process
   • We do not completely understand the science of pain
   • An intact brain is required for humans to experience suffering with pain
   • All humans experience pain – it is adaptive, has "message" and "meaning"

   2. How the normal brain experiences pain

   • In fibromyalgia the normal process of pain/symptom production is deranged
   • Research shows abnormal activity in the brain
   • There appears to be an amplification of pain with exposure to painful stimuli
   • There are abnormalities in levels of peptides – chemicals that communicate between brain and body
   • When an intervention works to reduce fibromyalgia pain, the brain appears to change

   3. The role of triggers in fibromyalgia

   • Physical, mental, emotional and environmental stressors may initiate the dysregulation
   • A single "event" or cumulative stressors may be identified
   • This fits the "neuro-plasticity model" for chronic pain production

II. The role of the sensitive temperament

- The work of Elaine Aron, PhD, and the "highly sensitive person"
- David Kiersey's "Idealist" temperament, the opposite of the cultural prototype
- Even without triggers, the tension created by being sensitive in a relatively insensitive culture may be sufficient to create dysregulation.
- The sensitive temperament requires periods of no and low stimulation in order to achieve homeostasis (health and balance)

III. Prevailing Myths about Fibromyalgia

- Inflammation
- Unhealed trauma
- Bad biomechanics
- Bad psychology

IV. Treating Fibromyalgia

I. Why so many "western" treatments fail

- Treatment will be unsuccessful if it does not change the brain
- The sensitive temperament needs to be taken into account

2. Why we are using a mind/body/spirit approach

- Other healing traditions support this approach
- Research into some of these interventions demonstrates brain changes

- There are no side effects
- Approaching the "problem" any other way is not "big enough"

3. How Complementary Medicine interventions work

- With a change in thought patterns (cognition) there is a change in the electrochemical flow of energy in the brain from the limbic system to the neo-cortex
- EFT (and certain other techniques) help to uncouple the electrochemical flow of energy between the limbic system and the hypothalamus

An Energy Psychology Definition of Chronic pain

In Traditional Chinese Medicine, the source of acupuncture, the heart is called the 'King' of the organs. The Internal Medicine Classic states: 'The heart commands all of the organs and viscera, houses the spirit, and controls the emotions.' In Chinese, the word for 'heart' (hsin) is also used to denote 'mind'. When the heart is strong and steady, it controls the emotions; when it is weak and wavering, the emotions rebel and prey upon the heart-mind, which then loses its command over the body.

What we call chronic pain is an interruption in a particularly sensitive person's electrical system resulting from emotional trauma. Repeated experiences of stress or trauma can cause the energy system to become disrupted and the flow of life force restricted, limiting our access to our capacity to think and act and make choices. If we repress the emotions (sadness, anger, fear) that arise in response to our traumatic experiences, the electrical system disruption will eventually show up as pain and dis-ease in the body. Clearing the disruption can clear the pain and change thought.

A Psycho-Spiritual Definition of Chronic pain

Chronic pain is obstructed spiritual energy reflected as pain in the body. One could call it "a sadness of the heart." Spirit is the best in us, our portal to all that is good and hopeful. Some of the essential qualities of spirit are love, expansiveness, generosity, creativity, imagination, possibility, openness, growth, flow and purpose. A sensitive person can be extraordinarily in tune with her or his spiritual qualities, but may feel unable to fully express them in what appears to be a harsh, critical, wounding world. As a result of traumas, a sensitive person may develop chronic pain from an emotional response to a limiting belief around which their whole being seems to constrict: "I can't express what I really feel, I can't be who I really am, I am not good enough. In order to matter or have significance in the world, in order to have inner peace, and in order to justify taking care of myself, I must remain ill." In a non-logical, unconscious intuitive way, this is a self-protective approach. Changing beliefs and choices can free the spirit and heal the body.

Using EFT for Freedom from Chronic Pain

These are the themes in this book:

- **Introduction** - Clearing and Calming Chronic Pain
- **Mapping the Healing** - Letting a Caged Spirit Fly Free
- **Mending a Broken Heart:** Healing and Re-Empowering a Sensitive Temperament

Even though my heart feels heavy and tight and sad, I honor myself for how hard this has been, I understand, and I even forgive myself. I was doing the best I could. I choose to love and appreciate and honor this powerful, world changing soul quality that I have been so blessed with.

- **Reframing Sensitivity**

Even though I worry that I am too sensitive, I want to deepen and expand my sensitivity in powerful wonderful ways. I choose to accept it as an honor, and learn how to share what I know in ways that are helpful.

- **Open the Cage of Anger and Pain**

Even though I am sad and mad and hurting all over, I know I deserve better. I don't have to be a volcano to stand up for myself.

- **Open the Cage of Fear**

Even though it doesn't feel safe to be me, I can re-invest my emotional inheritance of negative beliefs and expectations. I am choosing to focus on the essence of me, my strength, my largest vision of myself.

- **Open the Cage of Feeling Invisible**

Even though I had no voice and it wasn't safe or possible to say what I really thought, or speak up for myself, I honor myself for how hard that was, I love and accept myself, and I say YES to me!

- **Open the Cage of Overwhelm**

Even though I get overwhelmed, and I think I have to just soldier on and tough it out, I love and accept who I really am, as someone who likes things quiet and clear. I want to honor my deep inner strength and my goodness.

- **I am Eager to Please**

Even though I look for approval in all the wrong places, and I don't know how to connect with others without drowning and losing myself, I know now I don't have to *take care of somebody else to be OK. I honor my deep need for connection and meaningful relationships. I make creating and maintaining a good and satisfying relationship with **myself** my first priority.*

- **Open the Cage of "I'm Never Enough"**

Even though I thought that what I do had to Be Perfect, and I would have killed myself rather than admitting I was "weak," I honor my appreciation for doing things well, I am learning to open to the strength INSIDE me, and I am learning to trust the process.

- **The Positive Intention of Chronic Pain**

Even though I think if I get better there will be too many expectations of me, and people will have too much access to me, and then I will let people down, and a part of me thought I couldn't be "good" unless I was suffering, I am choosing to learn a new way of being with my body. I have a mission to bring peace to the world.

I choose the mission of bringing peace into my own life.

Chapter 2:
Mapping the Healing
Letting a Caged Spirit Fly Free

As I taught the Freedom from Fibromyalgia classes with Dr. Nancy Selfridge, I began to develop a way of tracking and visualizing the information I was gathering. It evolved into an image in my mind that I could keep track of on paper as well, and it helped me to see the person's whole experience all at once.

When I tap with someone, I now have all the information I need right in front of me. I can combine various parts of it, creatively sparking my intuition. Often I come up with a new idea or insight that surprises and delights me, or the client does, and this makes our work together even more interesting and fun.

I think of this diagram as the structure of beliefs and experiences and feelings that holds the illness in place. I notice that having the illness can serve a powerful purpose in a person's life: *Having pain, even disability, for some people, makes it possible for them to be in the world with more power and presence than they thought they could have had otherwise.*

Ask the question, "*What positive purpose does this illness serve in your life?*"

This question is bound to elicit puzzled looks at first, and a client's earnest insistence that they want nothing more than to be free of this condition. But eventually the light begins to dawn. The person begins to realize that having fibromyalgia or chronic fatigue, or another debilitating condition, is somehow keeping them safe, or allowing them to say NO when they don't feel capable or worthy of setting those boundaries themselves. Or the illness makes it possible for them to spend their time doing what *they* want to do, rather than meeting someone else's expectations – the "should's." Often this involves taking classes, reading self-help books, meditating, doing yoga, walking in the woods.

I will always remember the minister's wife in one of my classes who said, "If I didn't have fibromyalgia, I would have to *be* the minister's wife." Being a sensitive person, she was very shy and didn't like being in groups. It was very painful for her to "be" The Minister's Wife, and with fibromyalgia, she didn't have to! "Also, if I healed," she added thoughtfully, "I'd have to really deal with our relationship. This way I don't have time or attention to think about that."

You might imagine this diagram as an inner circle, a kind of cage of memories and beliefs and feelings and symptoms that holds the person's expressive spirit prisoner. There are various stations along the circle, for aspects of the problem. You would include a memory that brings you pain when you think about it, feelings, symptoms and behaviors, and negative beliefs about yourself that arose from that early (or recent) experience. The feelings and symptoms are seen as messengers that are trying to get your attention. Those messengers carry a positive purpose.

Letting a Caged Spirit
Fly Free

The positive purpose opens out to an outer circle, a more expansive view of what is possible, as if the cage door has opened and some inner part that had been cramped inside is allowed to step forth and breathe and move.

Here you can make decisions and choices based on what actually feels right or interesting or fun for you personally, instead of following someone else's rules. Here is the deeper truth about you. And when you think back through your life, you notice that this wonderful quality has been active in you all your life. It is who you really are! Now you can point yourself in a healing direction, guided by what feels right.

I described this map of the structure of healing chronic pain in my book, *The 8 Master Keys to Healing What Hurts* (available on my website, www.IntuitiveMentoring.com). This is an excerpt from Chapter 4, "The 8 Master Keys":

This is the map that we will use to calm and clear chronic pain (or any issue).

This map is a recipe for gathering information that you can use for yourself or your clients. Take an issue in your life, and respond to what comes up in each of the following eight aspects of it. Gather all your relevant memories, thoughts, symptoms, feelings, and beliefs.

14

Become aware of the Positive Purpose of these Inner Messengers.

Create tapping routines. Do a little or a lot each day. You can't OD on EFT. (Make sure you have a life though!) You can't do this wrong. It is helpful to work with a practitioner, but there is a lot that you can do on your own. Begin with the intention that you will transform your limited thinking into expansive thinking

I call the deepest most powerful truth about us "Wealth-Being."

• Wealth: The origin of the word means: Well-being, prosperity, happiness, wellness. As a old word it appears in language before 900 AD.

• We think of *having* wealth. We wish we had more of it. It always seems elusive. "They" get to "have" wealth, not little old me.

• What could it mean to BE wealth??

• Where in your life are you wealthy?
(wealthy = well, happy, prosperous)

• Where are you poor?

• All poverty is the result of caging the human spirit. Poverty is not just economic. Pain, depression, anxiety, fear, shame, worry, anger – all of this is poverty.

15

• How did we get into the cage of poverty thinking? Better question: How do we get ourselves out? Our healing is in our own hands, with EFT.

The 8 Master Keys to Healing What Hurts and Creating Wealth-Being:

Free your S-P-I-R-I-T-E-D Self

S – *Tap to reframe your* **Sensitivity.** Have you ever been told, "Oh, you are just too sensitive! What is wrong with you?" Learn what is **profoundly good** about being so sensitive. (Probably everyone with a chronic condition has a Highly Sensitive Temperament. Chapter 3 of this book is about being sensitive. The effects of this temperament is woven throughout all of these chapters.)

P – *Tap away the effects of* **Painful** *experiences from the past.* Life, especially your childhood, may have led you to believe that: You don't deserve to get what you want. It is not safe to be visible or heard.

I – *Tap to reframe the limited* **Identity** *you took on as a result* (beliefs).

- There is something wrong with me.
- It was my fault.
- My needs aren't important.
- I have to be ill in order to get what I need.

- I have to save the world *so that/before I can be safe.*

R – *Tap away the* **Responses** *in your body to this limited identity (caged spirit).* You couldn't express what you really felt, so you swallowed it, and now it is expressing as:
- pain in your body
- chronic illness
- sabotaging behavior, like avoidance, addictions, procrastination

I – *Tap for the deeper positive* **Intention** *of the symptoms and emotions.* But deep inside you that anger or pain is really a message to you, wanting you to know that:

- I can stand up for myself, express my own truth, ask for what I want.
- I deserve to take care of myself without feeling guilty!
- It is safe to be visible and be heard.

T – *Tap for knowing that the* **Truth** *about me is that I was born good!* (and, surprise, your goodness has always been there!) The Truth about you is that your Wealth-Being is good for the world!

- I belong here.
- I am called to be here; I have a purpose here.
- I deserve to prosper!
- My truth has always been in everything I have done.

17

E - **Evidence** *that you have always been this truth.* Find the examples of it in your life.

D - Set your **Direction.** Understand your own personal "Yum and Yuck meter". (Everything comes down to "Yum and Yuck".)

- Learn how to know What is Right for You.
- I deserve to take care of myself without feeling guilty!
- Tap into your own guidance.

SELF - Be Self - ish!

- It is safe to be visible and be heard.
- I am worthy of growing both spiritually and materially.
- Tap to feed your own soul. If *you* don't, no one will.

S-P-I-R-I-T-E-D SELF.

- We are all in this together.
- The healing that you accomplish benefits all of us!
- Free Your Caged Spirit!
- Tap into Your Wealth being!

I created this mnemonic of SPIRITED SELF so you could remember the aspects more easily. As you read the book, you will see that they form a Map. The inner shape holds the constricted poverty thinking. This is the structure of the problem, what holds it in place.

As we work through **SPIRITED SELF**, that constricted inner shape of the chronic condition "out-frames" into Wealth-Being thinking.

Taken all together, this Map forms the structure of healing.

The out-framed part of the Map contains the key and powerful techniques for your own self-care. The principle behind them is that if you create this moment right now to be full of what you love and feel good about, as much as possible, and do that in each moment, when the future gets here it will be full of what you love.

The future is always getting here! In that sense, there is no future. Just the ever-unfolding present moment, moving in the DIRECTION that you are setting with your intention and self-talk about who you are and what is possible for you.

Each of these aspects is deeply evocative. You could take each one in turn and explore it with your own thoughts and emotions, tapping with EFT for what comes up for you.

Another way to use this Map is this: I like to begin with a feeling, a body symptom or behavior, or a limiting belief, whatever is showing up most insistently to get my attention. I fill that in on the Map, and proceed to work through the rest of the aspects.

It is important to select **ONE SPECIFIC** experience that was challenging or painful, and a very good idea to give it a title. Create the title out of the worst moment of the memory.

The title is important mostly as an information

space, a trigger. What counts is that when you think of it, you really **feel** a physical response inside. Even though your mind may want to get theoretical or explanatory or creative with this, or you may think "I'm no good at this", let your body have its say here. Go with what provokes the strongest response inside.

Rate the intensity of your inner response from 0 - 10, or however you like to assess the intensity.

When you have completed the Map, use everything on it in your tapping session, adding any thoughts, feelings or images that come up intuitively as you go. You can re-use it as often as you like, until none of the stations on the Map bring up any negative thoughts or feelings.

Each of the other chapters in this book describes working with an emotional aspect of chronic pain. Since the Sensitive Temperament is the background of most chronic pain, I will talk about that first.

Chapter 3:

Mending A Broken Heart:

Healing and Re-Empowering a Sensitive Temperament

I have asked this question of many people: **"As a sensitive person, what concerns and issues do you want help with resolving?"**

Here is what one person said:

- Oh Lord, this is where I need the help. I have all of the characteristics of Emotional Sensitivity—to the extreme. I would like to know **how to deal with my extreme emotional sensitivity**. My mother always says, 'don't cry, it doesn't do any good. I could be crying all of the time.' I have been unemployed since August. I would complain to the CEO about my coworkers, and ended up being terminated.

- I easily **attach to people** - especially men - and have a hard time letting go.

- I hate **loud people** (my sister-in-law drives me crazy) and being in **chaotic places,** yet cannot keep my own home from being chaotic.

• I hate being so **overly sensitive** and I **take everything to heart,** and it remains there for a very, very, very long time.

• I am easily hurt, I suffer from depression - sometimes based on something someone has said or done to me. I am very prone to stimulus overload - loud noises, large noisy crowds, exhaust me.

• I often **feel like a total failure and disappointment** to everyone - including myself.

• I **feel like an outsider** - always on the outside looking in; I feel like I don't belong.

• **I want to be happy and I want to love myself** – however, I don't know where to find those things within me.

• I have been told I have psychic abilities and that I am a Light Worker - I'm **extremely intuitive** and am accurate on the things I feel - but sometimes I feel as if I've lost that intuitiveness. I've been asking God and the Angels for assistance for quite some time but feel as though I'm not being heard, or at least I'm not hearing them.

Each of these statements would make an excellent EFT set-up. The next step would be to think of particular, specific experiences in your life, especially as a child, when something happened that made you feel and think this way about yourself. Tap for all the different aspects of this experience until you no longer have the same response to that particular experience.

EFT is a wonderful tool for sensitive people. It can focus right in on the experiences that have hurt us so deeply, and dissolve both the pain and the beliefs we came to have about ourselves as a result. The more specific we can be with EFT, the more likely it is that we will have good results.

Painful Experience: A powerful memory that lies frozen in the past.

Most of us don't have any problem coming up with painful memories! But we tend to blame ourselves for what happens to us. We think, 'I am *too* sensitive! There must be something wrong with me. I should be able to just let this roll off my back!'

As a highly sensitive person myself, I have done my best over the years to reframe this quality as a gift. It IS a gift. The world needs what we have to offer!

My books (http://www.intuitivementoring.com/EFTbooks.html) are all about how to use EFT to heal the wounds of your sensitive nature so that you are empowered to use your gifts in the service of yourself, your family, your community and the world itself.

Here is an excerpt from my book on healing chronic pain with EFT, **The 8 Master Keys to Healing What**

Hurts:

If you are feeling overwhelmed by what is going on in your life and how you feel about it, and you can't even begin to think of where to start with EFT, these powerful and evocative questions will help you to be specific:

- What broke your heart?
- When did something die in you, or get blocked, or shut down?

Write out or tape yourself talking about your experiences. Then take each of the sentences of your story or journal entry that carries a charge for you, and turn it into a tapping sequence.

- Go deeper. *What did I lose as a result?*

A painful experience can make us feel that we have lost our sense of connection, belonging, safety, peace, joy, integrity, wholeness.

Tap for this deep loss. Add words to the second part of the EFT set-up that express your honoring of yourself for how hard this has been, and that you understand, and even forgive yourself. You have always been doing the best you could. Add some 'I choose' phrases. What inner state of being would you like to choose instead of how you had been feeling?

Here are some mores evocative questions that will help you get closer to the key experiences in your life that are asking for healing:

- What does this current event or feeling remind me of?
- If I could live life over again, what person or event would I prefer to skip?
- When was the last time I cried, and why?
- Who/what makes me angry, and why?
- What is my biggest sadness or regret?
- What is missing to make my life better?
- Three fears I would rather not have:
- What do I wish I had never done?

Your answers to these questions will help you to find specific experiences and aspects to tap for.

Ashe's Story: *I feel like a small child frozen in fear.*

Ashe took one of my group coaching series on healing the hurts that come from having a sensitive nature, and she had bravely volunteered to be a tapping demonstration subject. Since her tapping sessions over the weeks seemed quite profound and useful to her, I asked later if she would write a little about her background, and how the class had affected her. Her answer demonstrates the power of what happens to us as children, and how it shapes our adult behavior.

I am so grateful for her willingness to share this, and as always, honored when someone offers their story. These tales of pain and transformation become a guiding light for the healing of all of us.

"I don't want to be like my mother, and I am so much like her it's not funny.

"I feel like a small child frozen in fear. My mother was a teacher who always played the teacher. Whatever I wanted to do, she always said I was too young. To any of my child wisdom she would say in a derogative tone, 'What would you know? You're only a child,' even though I was proved right time and time again. I've cleared heaps around her with EFT, but nothing seems to touch this fear of doing what I am drawn to and love doing, and my fear of 'standing alone.'

"I started numbing my feelings

"That violent crazy side of her has terrified me and what it boils down to is I'm terrified of both doing and being, because I don't want to be like her. That started when I was very little. So I started being like my dad, which was controlling, numbing the feelings, effectively not-being. Appearing calm on the outside at all costs, because otherwise she'd 'get you' energetically once she started, and then you'd end up being wrong and punished, and the 'whipping post' for her to vent on.

"It required a huge amount of control not to respond, because I was so sensitive and felt all that so much. Until very recently I always got scared around overdoing things and being tired, because I would lose my patience (read shutting down, steely tolerance, and jaw-locking self-control). When I was little, reacting meant being shamed big time.

"This whole thing obviously touched off something in her that scared her too, because she couldn't deal with my reaction. Whenever I was angry she told me I was tired. The result was that by the time I was a teenager I got glandular fever and ended up permanently tired - until I started clearing my anger.

"An incident with her when I was much smaller (age 2 to 3) came up where she 'lost it ' and it was so terrifying that I disappeared. It was as if all there was, was her raging terror. I can see from my perspective now, that this was a frozen moment of raging fear that has been passed down the generations in my family for who knows how long. I am the first to acknowledge it, let alone deal with it. My grandmother got Alzheimer's rather than deal with her version of it.

"Yesterday I felt very edgy, and without knowing why, I started picking on my husband and getting really angry with him. I was watching it too. At that point I started to notice how scared and unreasonable I was being, and "I started to pay even more attention.

"I asked for grace to open my heart.

"It was as if a cold bony hand was gripping the inside of my stomach. I realized that having this fear and anger feeling inside herself was exactly what had made my mother pick on me and tell me all the horrible things that were wrong with me. So again, all I could do in that moment was surrender it and ask for grace to open my heart to myself and her.

"I noticed some time back that I could only use my energy in defiance. That wasn't how I wanted to do things any more, but I had no way of being with ease.

"All my inner knots are unraveling nicely now as fast as I can process, and your course and EFT have helped immensely. Things just popped out so easily. It was really such a great help to work from a different perspective. I felt very safe with you.

"So this is about where I'm up to, a bit dazed by the whole thing, but open to a new way of being and doing things, that I know is already waiting for me to be ready and open to it.

Healing and Re-empowering
a Sensitive Person:

• Painful experiences are felt more deeply by a sensitive person, especially as a child.

• Painful experiences lead to beliefs about who we are and what is possible for us in life.

• It may not be possible or safe to express the powerful anger, sadness, and fear, and shame that we feel during and after these painful experiences.

• Those feelings get 'stuffed' or swallowed.

• These stuffed feelings show up later in our lives as physical and emotional pain and illness.

• The people in our families who mistreated us did so because this is how they had been treated, and these were the beliefs and feelings they themselves took on.

• The tendency to replicate these beliefs and feelings and illnesses gets passed on down through the generations of a family.

• The fear of confronting the powerful feelings stops us from beginning a healing journey.

• Our personal healing can heal the whole family history.

Healing our family's history is on the way to healing the world! We just thought we had to **start** with healing the whole world, so that it would be a safe place for us. That was pretty exhausting.

Ashe's experience is a good illustration of how EFT can calm and clear the frozen anger and fear from incidents in our past - the source of much of the current physical pain in a sensitive person.

Chapter 4:
Reframing Sensitivity

Even though *I worry that I am too sensitive, I want to deepen and expand my sensitivity in powerful wonderful ways. I choose to accept it as an honor, and learn how to share what I know in ways that are helpful.*

Have you ever heard (or said about someone else):

- "Oh, you are just too sensitive!"
- "You take things so hard!"
- "Just let it roll off your back."
- "Why can't you just let it go!"
- And maybe even, "What's wrong with you? You are such a cry baby!"

You probably thought they were right - there must be something wrong! Being sensitive is an actual emotional temperament. I believe it is the kind of awareness that can save the world.

I speak as a "highly sensitive person" myself. It has taken me most of my life to understand this temperament and value it for its gifts. I have worked with many people who are extra sensitive to stress, traumatic experiences, and environmental toxins.

People with this temperament are also extraordinarily sensitive to beauty and spirituality, and

© *Rue Hass 2008   IntuitiveMentoring.com*
Profoundly light -hearted strategies for unsticking stuck stuff

they all have a desire to be a good custodian of the earth. If you're reading this and feeling, "Yeah, that's me, all right!", YOU are the help that is on the way, whether you are sensitive yourself, or partnered/ working with/ interacting with/or the parent of someone who is sensitive.

Listen to **Dr. Nancy Selfridge** on the Highly Sensitive Temperament and chronic pain:

"I believe that chronic pain patients start out with a sensitive system to begin with - by birthright - temperamentally. One of the tests that I have administered in my practice is the Highly Sensitive Person test developed by Elaine Aron. All my patients scored high on this. And the other thing that I noted, if I asked my patients if they'd done a Myers-Briggs temperament inventory they were, except for two patients in my recollection, they were Intuitive Feelers. The I or E, the P or J doesn't matter so much but that NF function seems to identify a nervous system that has fewer filters on it than is considered the norm.

"One of the things both Rue and I try to do in our work, is help people understand that it is okay to honor the sensitive temperament in order to be well. The literature says that people who are wired this way need periods of no and low stimulation in order to achieve homeostasis.

"What is the difference between people who are highly sensitive and get fibromyalgia and people who are highly sensitive and don't? I don't know.

"That's fascinating. One of my observations is, my friends who are highly sensitive who have not gotten sick have made dramatically different lifestyle choices than I did. That's one. And some people have somehow gotten enough recognition, perhaps early in life, that it sort of fortified them against the slings and arrows of normal fortune, much less outrageous fortune.

"So how do the interventions work when they do if we use energy therapy? I believe when we change our thought patterns we're going to see change in electrochemical flow in our brain from the limbic system. We can use some cognitive approaches but we also can manipulate subtle energies. I think Energy Psychology techniques help to uncouple old established patterns that are translated into pain in our patients, and into autonomic dysfunction.

"Patients ask me, how does this work? I tell them it is sort of like running the defrag program on your computer. Whatever happened to you that triggered this real problem in your brain and over activated this area in your brain - this area is sort of chaotic and fragmented with the information in there. When we do EFT it is like running a good defrag. That seems to be a model that probably is not very accurate, but it works.

"It has become apparent to me that chronic pain patients are like "canaries in the coal mine" responding to our stressful culture and environment with real illness and debilitation. There is nothing about this that is fictitious, nor evidence of psychological disease or bad character. This disorder demands an expansion of our understanding of stress and disease.

"As my own awareness of the multiple stressors we are exposed to increases, I expand my counseling of my sensitive patients to include diet and nutrition to avoid inflammation and illness, supplements to correct nutritional deficiencies and diligent counseling about stress management strategies and interventions.

"Most of all, I give permission to patients to live for their own hearts' desires, to explore their limiting beliefs and to honor their sensitive temperaments. It is this latter path that will best help the sensitive soul from becoming sick again."

(Dr. Nancy Selfridge, from transcript of presentation at Association for Comprehensive Energy Psychology Conference, May, 2005)

So let's get started!

Any kind of chronic pain - whether physical, emotional or mental - is about what we believe about our experience. Limiting beliefs create a disruption in the body's energy field.

Learn and use EFT to neutralize these limiting beliefs.

Starting with the Karate Chop point or the Sore Spot, use the following EFT setups.

Even though...

- I worry that I am **TOO** sensitive
- I feel so deeply
- I am so open to others' emotions
- I am easily hurt and upset
- I don't like conflict
- It's hard to stop feeling sad sometimes
- I can't watch the news or sad or violent movies
- I get depressed easily
- I get overwhelmed

I deeply and completely love and accept myself

Even though...

- I can't stand large crowds
- I can't take loud noise

- I don't like hectic environments
- I wish I were tougher and could let things roll off easier
- I think my sensitivity is a weakness
- I think something is wrong with me. It is my fault.
- I wish things didn't bother me so much
- I wish my emotions weren't so obvious to other people
- I wish I could let things go and not worry so much
- I hide my sensitivity from others

I deeply and completely love and accept myself

Now Break out of The Cage of the P.A.S.S.T. (Pain, Anger, Sadness, Stress, Trauma) this way:

1. What have people said to you about your sensitivity?

- Tap on: Even though people have said _____ , I deeply and completely love and accept myself

2. How has that made you feel? Where do you feel it in your body?

- Tap on the feelings and emotion in your body

3. What did you come to believe about yourself as a result?

- Tap on the beliefs.

4. Choose a specific disturbing incident from your life connected with being sensitive.

- Make a movie or inner story of the specific incident. Give it a title.
- Note details: clear, fuzzy, movement, still, sound, silent, etc.

NOW TAP:

Tap on the title:

Even though I have this _____ (title) _____ story in my body about being sensitive, I deeply and completely love and accept myself.

- Tap while you watch and feel the story unfold.
- Tap on the worst parts.
- Tap on all the aspects.
- Note what has changed after you tap.

Celebrate your sensitivity!

Turning Problems into Preferences

Use EFT to enhance, expand, enlarge and deepen your gifts!

Let's start with that tapping list that framed all the problems we experience from our sensitivity, and RE-frame them as our gifts. Then we can make them even better!

Now, the following words are mine. *You* find better ones, ones that fit *you* and feel good to *you*! Maybe you like to speak in superlatives - use those. Maybe you have more profound or more spiritual ways of expressing what is truly the best and loveliest and greatest about you – go for it! Use your best words - ones that make you light up inside!

Tap using the normal EFT spots. But instead of saying "Even though..." try saying "Especially because..."   Take out the old phrases in parentheses below and replace them in each case with what follows:

Especially because (*I worry that I am TOO sensitive*)

I LOVE that I am so sensitive. I choose to deepen and expand my sensitivity in powerful wonderful ways.

Especially because (*I feel so deeply*)

I have this fabulous capacity to feel deeply. **I choose**

to accept it as an honor, and learn how to share what I know in ways that are helpful.

Especially because *(I think my sensitivity is a weakness)*

I like that I am sensitive. **I choose** to love and appreciate and honor this powerful, world changing soul quality that I have been so blessed with. The world needs what I have to offer! I am ready to be more!

Especially because *(I think something is wrong with me. It is my fault)*

I believe that I am a good person. **I choose** to open to what I know in my deepest heart that I can become! I love and appreciate and honor this precious being that I am!

Especially because *(I wish things didn't bother me so much)*

I am glad that I am so aware. **I choose** to trust the Universe to handle the problems and I use my awareness and my energy to make a difference in this world that I care so much about.

Continue tapping *beginning with the phrase* **"Especially Because [EB]:"**

EB...*I have this wonderful gift of being able to think and speak in abstract big picture, profound concepts*

I choose to deepen and strengthen my ability to be an Imagineer, and use my manifestation ability even better so that the goodness I sense has a space to live in, in this world.

EB...*being cooperative and diplomatic is important to me*
I choose to break the rules that aren't working for me and make new ones that feel right, in ways that still honor other peoples' integrity and intentions

EB...*I hunger for deep and meaningful relationships*
I make creating and maintaining a good and satisfying relationship **with myself** my first priority.

E.B...*I value personal growth, authenticity and integrity*
I choose to discover my own strengths and excellence, and do everything I can to enlarge them.

EB ...*I am internally deeply caring*
I choose to take just as good care of myself as I do of _____.

EB...*I am deeply committed to the positive and the good*
I choose to honor that commitment to myself!

EB...*I have a mission to bring peace to the world*
I choose a mission of bringing peace into my own life.

EB...*I have a strong personal morality*
I choose to stand even taller in my own strong life!

EB...*I often make extraordinary sacrifices* for someone/
something I believe in
I choose MYSELF!!!!

EB...*I have a good imagination*
I choose to find amazing ways of bringing magic
into my life where there was only misery before!
Evolution itself depends on how good I get at this!

EB...*I think I am unusual and unique*
I choose to stand up for myself and express who I
am with love and a light heart. No one can resist that...

*Of course, you are noticing that you don't have
to apply these phrases ONLY to the issues of
sensitivity!*

Chapter 5 :

Open The Cage of Anger and Pain

Even though *I am sad and mad and hurting all over, I know I deserve better. I don't have to be a volcano to stand up for myself!*

Any time you feel angry or irritated, it is connected to your inner life and your entire history by a fine web of associations that lead right back into your childhood, and beyond. In fact, you could say that the little incident that got your attention is the latest manifestation of a story that has been repeated in the lives of your ancestors in some way for many generations.

So, think of some pain that you have, physical or emotional. Now think of a recent time when you were angered or irritated by something going on in your life. Maybe the connection between the event and the body symptoms and your behavior is obvious, and maybe not. In any case, this is the corner of the fishing net that we will pull on to find out what is caught in it.

Much of the following material comes from clients who have sent me their thoughts about anger and pain, in the context of our working together to calm and clear the pain and anger from their energy field.

Here are the words of one woman's pain and anger story

"A list of what has showed up in me over time as symptoms: migraines, headaches, menstruation problems, face pain, pain in the muscles in my cheeks, my teeth hurt, my jaw hurt. Neck, arm, joints from lymph. There has been pain in my stomach, back, and butt. When I have been sitting too long, my legs and calves grip up on me. My feet used to hurt a lot, but that is not too bad now. I have had problems sleeping, irritable bowel syndrome, loss of libido. I have a very sensitive temperament and sensitive body.

"I feel that my body is betraying me. It is not cooperating. There are things I want to do and it is not cooperating. I am angry at my body!

"My brother is married to a woman with two exceptionally talented daughters. My older sister had a beautiful voice. I was invited to her performance to hear her sing. She was amazing.

"My brother was going on and on and on about her. I thought, "If I don't get out of this room I am going to start screaming!" I had to leave. I was thinking, "Why in hell did you never encourage me? Never recognize me?" No one in my family encouraged me to do anything. I can sing too! My brothers were the gods in my family. They got everything!

"I felt such anger and grief. I was in tears all the way home. This should have been me! Like I'm getting my nose rubbed in this. I will never again be able to go out and see her sing. Or see anyone in my family getting recognition.

"When I kept a list of all the things I was angry about, to tap on, my anger list was very long.

"And then I am angry at myself for being angry!

"I finally quit my job last year because I was angry at my boss ALL the time. It put my family in a terrible financial situation. If she hadn't been such a horrible manager, I could have put up with the job. I wrote a scathing letter to her. I felt better for a while. Of course, I never mailed it.

"I have anger at myself for not having figured out how to let go of my anger. I am sad that I am sad. I have to be careful, thinking I have no right to be angry and sad any more. Now, I feel guilty if I am not happy and blissful that I am not in that job. I feel like I have to be up and happy and chipper for my husband.

"It made me angry that I couldn't tough it out. I should be able to do this job. Not being able to tough it out would be a failure in my family, a sign of weakness. I should be able to let it roll off, not let it bother me.

"That is a philosophy l I was raised with. If you got hurt: 'Oh you're not that bad, just tough it out.' I didn't tell my dad I had quit my job because he would see me as a failure.

"Now, after the work we have done, and all the tapping, I know in my heart that the failure would have been to stay in that job.

"One of the hardest things about this healing work is that it really is hard work. It is asking people to REALLY look at their injuries and wounds. You feel that pain again. I found the tapping could let me get rid of anger if I could focus on what it was the tapping helped me get rid of. Then I could let go of the anger. I can't explain it. It just makes you feel better.

"Getting rid of anger, I feel more relaxed. I hold anger tension in my body as a coiled spring. I can literally feel tenseness draining out of me and I can breathe and relax.

"The other thing that tapping really does for me is that phrase, "Even though...whatever, I deeply and completely love and accept myself." It has had a profound effect on my own sense of value. I have come to appreciate myself, recognize myself, my own intelligence. EFT gets that phrase into your belief system. It gets into your cells somehow."

If you have read my book, **The 8 Master Keys for Healing What Hurts**, you have read much of the amazing story of Leila, who has healed herself from fibromyalgia using EFT. Also, if you have seen the new short videos about EFT that are on the <u>www.emofree.com</u> website, she is there, talking about her success. I made her "Leila" in the book, but she gave me permission to share that Celia is her real name. Here is one of the things she wrote as we were dealing with anger:

"...More importantly - I have realized how much stronger my anger is towards my mother over awful things she did to **others** than it is over anything she did to me. You gently pushed me a bit to recall those feelings and I came up with almost nothing, - but huge rage over her treatment of others.

"Today I thought my way through to understanding that from a very young age I knew two things from my DAD! That I was a disappointment and that young 'soldiers' have to toughen up. So two things developed in me at the same time - an acceptance that I deserved to be thought poorly of, and a toughness to carry pain and 'keep my chin up" and not fight back against the commander - mom.

"My Dad's war experience cut him off from his own sensitivities, and he saw his children's frailties as weaknesses.

"So now I understand better why I have

trouble recalling my buried anger directly related to mom's treatment of ME.

"I thought I deserved it and that I had to learn to be tough.

"It wasn't until I was a teenager that I began to **feel** anger - but even that was mainly about mom's treatment of others.

"So the origins of my low self-esteem (and the fibromyalgia) are buried very, very deep. Whatever anger I may have felt and buried as a very young child was pushed down even further by the certainty that I was a bad girl and deserved (more than the other children) to be treated poorly - and that my ability to accept that treatment meant I was becoming a good little soldier.

"No wonder I have trouble recalling anger over how I was treated, but no trouble recalling anger over how the rest of my family was treated.

"That was so interesting to me just how blank I was when you asked me to specifically recall my own personal anger over how I was treated.

"I'm onto it now though, and will work on getting some tappable phrases figured out. Thank you. Thank you!"

Obviously writing the above email sparked her thinking, because a day later this email came:

"…However, this fibromyalgia is dug in deep. Talking to you last Wednesday really helped me uncover a whole new aspect, when I realized that the enormous anger I carry towards my mother is mainly related to her mistreatment of OTHERS. The anger I carry about her mistreatment of ME is buried much, much deeper.

"So why, why, why is that?? And ah - hah! I have finally uncovered my father's involvement!!

"By the way, I do fully understand that they were doing the best they could with what they had (their own wounded selves) and the damage they did was completely unintentional - just like me - and look at the unintentional damage I did!!!!!

"Yes, the lights are finally coming on here!!

"So, for fibromyalgia, it feels necessary to do the 'hard work in the trenches' even after having these mental breakthroughs. Do you find that to be generally true?

"Here are what I found to be tappable phrases about my father's involvement in my ability to stuff my anger way down deep into potential fibromyalgia territory. I haven't tapped on them yet, but when I do I'll let you know how it goes. I am so looking forward to breaking out of all this into the light - I know I'm already well on my way.

"So, the hard work part:

"Even though - (each of the below) - I deeply and completely love and accept myself and am open to healing the situation now.

• my dad treated me like I was a disappointment
• my dad treated me like a young soldier who had to toughen up
• my dad taught me to accept that I deserved to be thought poorly of
• my dad taught me how to be tough
• my dad taught me to keep my chin up and carry the emotional and physical pain
• my dad taught me not to fight back against mom
• my dad saw his children's frailties as weaknesses
• my dad's war experience cut him off from his own sensitivities
• I have trouble recalling my buried anger directly related to mom's treatment of ME
• I thought I deserved it and I had to be tough
• the anger I felt was pushed very far down inside
• the origins of the low self esteem are buried very deep
• the anger was pushed down by the certainty that I was a bad girl

- the anger was pushed down by the certainty that I deserved to be treated badly
- my ability to accept that treatment meant I was becoming a good little soldier, which won dad's silent approval

"Time to get to work on this."

Even though all that happened ... that doesn't make me a bad person!

Most of our EFT training is about what to say at the beginning of the set up phrase, but I find my heart and my imagination are always drawn to the second half of the equation.

In the second half of the set-up we are healing the future, supporting and honoring and welcoming our own presence in it. We are holding the "problem" differently within our energy field, and therefore inviting and allowing ourselves to be held differently in the whole as well. One of my clients got a lot of good results from adding the phrase: *"And that doesn't make me a bad person."* Let's use it!

Step Off the Beaten Path
Out of the Cage...

Care for Your Soul! Use all that freed up power to appreciate yourself, instead of beating yourself up!

Use these affirmations — or even better, make up your own!

- It is OK and safe to let myself experience that anger and *that doesn't make me a bad person*
- I am choosing to resist my usual story about this pain *and that doesn't make me a bad person either*
- *That doesn't make me a bad person.* These are just thoughts and I don't have to believe them
- *That doesn't make me a bad person* and I can go ahead and feel what I feel anyway
- I wish things were different *and that doesn't make me a bad person*
- I love and accept myself *enough* that my symptoms can go away now
- I love and accept myself *enough* that I can just feel the wrong-ness and be OK with that anyway
- I am doing the best I can
- We are all doing the best we can
- I honor myself for how hard this has been
- I can surrender what I thought I knew and open to a deeper truth about myself!
- I am a better person than I thought I was!
- Soldiering on and toughing it out is not required! Healing is OK!

© *Rue Hass 2008* IntuitiveMentoring.com
Profoundly light-hearted strategies for unsticking stuck stuff

Chapter 6:
Open The Cage of Feeling Invisible

Even though *I had no voice and I feel hurt and invisible, I love and accept myself and I say YES to me!*

Often in EFT sessions I ask people the question, *"What did you want to say that you couldn't?"* Here are four examples of tapping sessions that dealt with this question.

Example One:

I was listening as someone was telling me how much better she was doing since our last session. The pain and cramping that had made her hands "stuck closed" had loosened up now. But then she began to describe how the pain seemed to be *"moving up my arms into my neck, where it used to be, a sharp, burning pain."*

I asked her when she first started noticing pain like this, and she began talking about thirty years earlier when she had such terrible tension in her jaw.

I imagined her jaw clenched closed - and the question popped out. "What did you want to say back then, or even earlier in your childhood, but couldn't?"

The answer wasn't right on the surface for her yet.

Tapping on the side of her hand, she mused out loud until she got to it:

> "There was something in my mind all the time back then. I kept thinking, 'I can't wait to get out of childhood, I can't wait to get out of my family. I wanted to scream - Let me out of here!!! This is a crazy place. I don't belong here!' "
>
> "You know what?" she said, in surprise. "I was keeping my mouth closed so I wouldn't say that to my mother! And I wanted to say 'Why are you hitting me???' I had to control myself so I wouldn't ask 'Why?' when she said 'NO, you can't ride your bike, go for a walk, or play outside.' She always said 'NO.' And when I asked her why, she always said, 'Because I said so.' **I had no voice.**"

I had been scribbling furiously as she said all this, and now we had lots of set-up statements that cycled around *wanting and needing and having something to say, and not being able to say it.* She was easily able to make the connection with situations in her life ever since then, when she had something to say that was her own, but she didn't say it. In fact, she had only recently escaped from a marriage where she had no voice, and now found herself in a relationship where she could see herself falling into the same pattern, though she was now well beyond the helpless person she had been earlier in her life.

By the time we were done tapping, this woman who had been feeling waves of tension sweeping through and out of her jaw, found it was now relaxed and open. Now she could feel what she wanted to say to her current partner with strength and clarity.

Example Two:

Another time that I popped this question this week was when a different client was talking about the dreams she was having.

"Lately all my dreams have a theme of 'Pay attention to me,'" she said.

She was feeling as if there was a child part of her that she hadn't acknowledged, that there were **"feelings inside that I am not feeling - they are stuck in there."**

I asked her to just use her imagination and start talking. What could this be about? Often a person says they don't know what is going on, but when I say "Just pretend that you do know," they start talking and something almost always emerges that is a revelation for both of us.

In this case, this woman, who is about 35 and has a job that is OK but doesn't really tap into her creativity and intelligence, began to talk.

She said: *"Well, I have always had a hard time in my life knowing what I want to do. I am always carried along by others' expectations. **I feel scared of listening and finding out what I want.**"*

This last sentence jumped out at me.

Where in your body do you feel that "scared of finding out what I want" feeling, I asked? Often when we give our attention to something that we have been avoiding, it just naturally begins to open out. Giving our attention to the physically held aspect of the feeling is safer than approaching it directly as an emotion or memory.

"I feel it a lot in my throat - it's tight," she said. "It's tight. It is like there is a lot of heavy sadness stuck in my throat. **My throat is contracted around this sadness.** It wants to come up and out, but my throat doesn't want it to come out."

"What if you let it up and out?" I asked. "What would happen?"

"Oh, I would make a HORRIBLE sound - my head might explode - I couldn't control it!" she exclaimed.

We began our tapping right there, with the sensations in her throat and the sadness. To make this a safe experience for her, I invited my client to imagine that there was an ally in her own belief system - a real person, an angel, a mythical figure - that could hold her safely while she tapped, so that her throat could be opening. She had been reading Carolyn Myss' book about archetypes, and chose the Angel archetype as "a strong, serene, supportive presence that could guide me and protect me through it." I asked her to build an image of this presence, and how it felt to be held by it. Then we tapped.

She realized that this strong painful sadness came from feeling abandoned as a child. She had been holding this deep pain in since then. Her throat had been closed around the fear of feeling this pain. Now that she had been alerted by her dreams, and knew what they were about, she knew that she could handle working with the issue with EFT.

Example Three:

Another client called to say that she (it just happened that these examples are all women, but it could just as easily been men!) wanted to cancel the session because she had this terrible cough that was draining her energy. She felt exhausted all the time. She had actually had this cough for many years, she told me, but it was particularly bad right now. She had an appointment tomorrow to see a doctor about her hypothyroidism.

Instead of canceling, we worked on the cough.

"What are you trying to cough up?" I was thinking. Right away I asked my question. Her answer turned up something interesting. Her issues came down to this:

"I didn't have any right to have an opinion, even though I knew inside that my opinion was right. My mother punished me for saying what I thought if I disagreed with her. But when I think of it, my grandmother never was able to say, or even know, what she thought. This issue must go way back in my family."

Long story short here, it turns out that in naturopathic medicine, the thyroid reflects a person's voice in their life. When the voice "feels trapped," over time, the accumulated effect gives rise to symptoms that can include poor thyroid function. It makes sense that holding in and repressing one's own truth could result in physiological symptoms like:

- severe fatigue, loss of energy
- weight gain, difficulty losing weight
- depression and depressed mood
- joint and muscle pain, headaches

We tapped on her cough. We tapped on several specific events in her life around the time that the cough began to show up, where she had felt that someone was trying to "kill me emotionally," and she hadn't felt able to speak up for herself. It wasn't too long before she said, *"Now I know I have a right to see things my way, and I have a right to have an opinion!"*

Example Four:

One more example of several. I guess the universe has been on a roll here to get my attention! I think I will begin asking this question of everyone.

Another client, Patsy, had also been telling me how much better she is doing lately. "My self talk is much more reassuring," she was saying. I asked her for some examples.

"My self talk says: 'Slow down. Do one thing at a time. Do what you can do. You don't have to do it all right now.'

"I am slower to get annoyed or irritated with myself. I understand myself better now. The only thing I am not so good at is letting go of all the Shoulds.

"In fact, it has been kind of a big plus for me to have the disease I do." (*She has* Crohn's Disease.)

Now, statements like Patsy's last one are a huge red flag for me! To me they mean that some body condition has become part of the client's identity, and is performing a function for them that, inside, they think they can not perform for themselves, for whatever reason. The equation goes like this:

Physical condition = sabotage of healing in order to protect myself.

I asked Patsy what she meant by "big plus." She said: *"If you eat wrong, or hold emotional things in, the disease flares up.* **It gives me power I don't have on my own to say 'no.'"**

"So, Patsy," I asked, "Who, in your past, could you not say 'no' to?"

"I couldn't say 'no' to my mother. Her routine was always 'Mother knows best.' She made my life miserable. I had a very close relationship with her when I was little, but the cost was in saying 'no' to me in order to say 'yes' to her. I tried, I argued with her, but that got me in a lot more trouble. It was just easer to give up, give in."

To work with this sabotaging set-up with Patsy, I mapped the information so it would all be right there in front of me as we tapped. You can create your own map. Think of some interesting and easy-to-remember shape that has several points, each of which can be a gathering place for certain information. I use a stick figure of the human body.

We chose a situation in Patsy's history that illustrated the problem with "saying no" and triggered a reaction to it in her body.

We gave the situation a **TITLE**:
Mother Knows Best

Under that I wrote her statement:

I had to say 'no' to me in order to say 'yes' to her.

The **FEELINGS AND EMOTIONS** were:

- anger
- discomfort
- sadness

These feelings get triggered by:

- the snide tone in her voice
- the look on her face

Translated into words they mean:

- You are so wrong
- I hate you for your choice
- You shouldn't want this.
- You should want what I want.

The **SYMPTOMS AND BEHAVIORS** were:

- a clenching feeling in my stomach and my chest that moves across my collarbone
- a feeling of bracing myself

- my shoulders feel like they are weighted down
- I am waiting for confidence to magically descend

I pointed out the interesting fact that the word "shoulders" has the word "should" in it, and there is the evocative play on words in "wait/weight," all of which can be woven creatively into the EFT wording.

The **BELIEFS** that arose from the experience were:

- I don't have a right to my own opinion
- What I think doesn't matter
- I have no power
- I am not good enough

The **POSITIVE INTENTION** of the emotions was:

- My anger and sadness want me to acknowledge that I am a person in my own right
- I am free to think for myself
- It is OK for me to want what I want
- I can express my own opinion and still be loved and supported
- *I can **say 'Yes'** to me!*

Together we tapped for all of these emotions, symptoms, and beliefs. For me, one of the good things about having all these words and phrases right in front of me in my map is that it stimulates my intuition and my creativity. I find myself riffing off of unusual combinations of these words and concepts in a way that is fun to do, and often funny. It is a good thing to laugh in the midst of a serious EFT session!

I concocted various takes on "Mother Knows Best" at one point, playing with:

- Mother No's Best...
- How good do YOU want to be at No-ing...
- The No's of Truth...
- Your own opinion is as clear as the No's on your face...
- I should **No** better...
- I **can and do** No **better** now!
- I can carry on my own shoulders what my Self Knows about my No's!
- Probably some even better ones are occurring to you right now.

We completed the tapping session by tapping in all the Positive Intentions. I used a similar creative weaving style, sometimes with humor, but more often with the intention of grounding Patsy's own sincere, powerful sense of Presence and Truth. Now, when she looks back on her life, Patsy can recognize that this sense of rightness and strength and trust in her self has been there always. I invited her to remember specific times where she could Notice that this is true. She has always had an opinion and a voice, and now she KNOWS she can trust it. *YES!*

Chapter 7:
Open The Cage of Fear

Even though it doesn't feel safe to be me, I can re-invest my emotional inheritance of negative beliefs and expectations. I am choosing to focus on the essence of me, my strength, my largest vision of myself. I have Great Expectations!

I have a friend who does healing work with her friend who has cancer.   She said this:

"My friend is Jewish and I am aware of the difficulty of her childhood, with two parents whose childhood was deeply scarred by the holocaust. I wonder if their child-rearing practices and the impact on my friend is a component of her cancer. I have thought of her work towards healing as generational work. I wonder about how the violence that her parent's generation experienced ripples out to other generations, how the history of violence that is so much a part of human history ripples out and is manifested as disease."

What did you expect?

I am powerfully fascinated by the emotional inheritance from our ancestors, and how that determines who we think we are and what we think we can expect of life.

Haven't we all heard: "You get what you expect!" And "Who do you think you are!"

What if we are even addicted to our expectations? There is increasing speculation and even scientific evidence that this is true.

Well, if we are going to be addicted, we might as well choose some good expectations to be stuck to, right? So why don't we just start out with a positive life view? Why do so many of us remember being sad as children, and now are sad - or angry - adults?

How do we get to an inner place of saying, "This is a false identity, not the true, healthy, me"?

What are YOU expecting? And - what makes you think that?

All of us who do EFT are, consciously or unconsciously, doing constant research on the effect of our expectations on our minds and bodies, and how to change them. Our tapping sends messages of healing and transformation across space and time.

I received this evocative, thoughtful email along these lines from my client Mischa (not her real name), a couple of weeks after her first session. I had invited her to share some of the reflections that arose in her after we did our work together.

What was going on when I was in the womb?

Mischa's email (all the words until the next headline are hers):

> "I wanted to share something with you that I read in your book that generated a powerful charge in me - enough to bring a big lump into my throat as I read it.

"This is the quote from your book:

'We are born into a family story about 'the way it is supposed to be.' So even in the womb, we are literally surrounded by and absorb the effects of our mother's family story in its effects on her body, mind, emotions and spirit at the cellular level of her body, our host. We feel the effects of our father's family story in our DNA, energetically, and in our mother's responses to him, even before our birth.' (**The 8 Master Keys to Healing What Hurts**)

"So what was going on when I was in the womb? Well, my mother had blood clots threatening her life and the doctors strongly urged her to have an abortion as the medication they had available to treat her wasn't safe during pregnancy. My mother obviously chose not to abort and all turned out well in the end, but what feelings must have flooded her - and me?

"What's more intense than literally having your life on the line? The fear - for her life, for mine, for what would happen to my four older siblings if anything happened to her. Maybe anger, that she should find herself in such a situation - and maybe sadness, for the same reason. I literally owe my life to my mother in more than a purely biological way.

"And my father. Childhood in wartime Europe, his own father away in the army, deported, literally seeing bodies floating down the Elbe River, ten years or so in the oppressive Communist regime in East Germany and two relocations following that.

"Life WAS about resigning oneself to harsh realities, hunkering down and surviving.

"What does it mean to be in survival mode?

- "It means you have to do what's necessary at the moment, regardless of how you feel."
- "It means you have to swallow feelings that don't serve necessity."
- "It might mean that you have to avoid attracting attention – 'keep a low profile.'"
- "It might mean that you have to avoid displeasing someone in power."
- **"It means IT'S NOT SAFE TO BE YOURSELF."**

"How much of my behavior was about who I really am and how much of it was about survival? Looking at it as objectively as one CAN look at oneself, I think it was both.

"Is that where the pattern formed of wanting so badly to make someone else happy? Is this the origin of my love/hate relationship with responsibility and meeting other people's expectations? I think there must be at least a connection for me to have felt such an emotional jolt when I read that paragraph in your book.

"I think there's a little girl part of me who still thinks there's a kind of equation I can benefit from: Make other people happy and THEN you can be yourself, because you'll have the love that you need. It's really about love.

"But if you think you have to earn love, then it is always in the background that YOU are not really loved, that it's the performance you're giving that's really garnering that praise and affection that you need.

Is it My Fault?

"I feel guilty because really, I know that my parents loved and do love me. There's a mountain of evidence that proves their love and good intentions. So how did I manage to take that niggle of insecurity out of it, along with many undeniably good things?

"Part of me thinks there must be something wrong with me to feel pain or angst in the first place."

The Truth of us

(Rue's voice now!) I suspect that all of our (often unconscious) obscuring beliefs, actions, positioning, and emotions flow from our emotional inheritance, the experience of our ancestors. All of our scramblings to survive distort the knowledge of our own sacred uniqueness, even - or maybe especially - from ourselves. We do this for all kinds of reasons, I think, but they all add up to not feeling able to be who we really are in the world safely.

But somehow, way behind our sense of unworthiness and hidden from view, especially our own, I believe there is actually a pure sense of our own perfection and radiant beauty. It is the blueprint for who each of us is in our own uniqueness. The distortion is like an identity that we are wearing. It is not the truth of us.

The Biology of Belief

In his book The Biology of Belief, Bruce Lipton tells a great story about a study done by the Baylor School of Medicine, published in 2002 by the New England Journal of Medicine. The surgeon doing the study was trying to figure out which part of the surgery he was performing for people with severe and debilitating knee pain was giving his patients relief.

In the first two groups, he did standard treatment procedures. In the third group he sedated the patient, talked and acted just like he would if he was doing the surgery, but didn't actually do anything, and then stitched the patient up. All three groups had the same post-op care. The third group was not told for two years that their surgery had been fake.

Amazingly (or maybe not), all three groups improved equally! One man, who was walking with a cane before the "fake surgery" now plays basketball with his grandchildren.

Obviously these people all expected to get better from surgery! But how much of their improvement had to do with the surgery? What we believe is true, is. What we expect will happen, does.

Create a magical tapping routine - for yourself, AND for your ancestors

I invite you to create a transformative EFT tapping routine for yourself. Pick out all the ideas and phrases in Mischa's letter and in my comments that struck you, and add ideas and phrases from your own experience. Also add what you know or guess about of your parents' experience, and your grandparents', and your great grandparents', and... Use your imagination.

Sometimes, begin your set up statements with "Especially because..." instead of "Even though". Notice what feels different when you do that.

Here are some examples:

Especially because I probably inherited my mother's fear - for her life, for mine - and **especially**

because I inherited her anger and her sadness that she should find herself in such a situation, **I am choosing to remember** my true story: that I am a sensitive, bold, bright, beautiful sovereign being who has been called here on purpose!... to be a source and force for love and goodness for myself that will flow from me as a blessing into the future.

> I love and accept myself and I know that I am safe now.

And **especially because** my father's life was about resigning himself to harsh realities, hunkering down and surviving, **I honor myself** for the conflicts that this has set up for me in my own life, and **I honor myself** for how hard that has been, and **I am choosing now** to change history! **I am choosing** to find ways to break free of those ancestral conflicts, and free myself to make decisions that support my deepest well being.

> I love and accept myself and I know that I am free now.

Especially because a part of me has thought that I have to earn love, and it is always in the background of my thoughts that I am not really loved, that it's the performance I'm giving that's really garnering that praise and affection that I need, **I accept** this part of me, **I accept** that it feels this way, and **I am choosing now** to focus on the blueprint of me, the essence of me carries all my strength, all my love, my largest vision of the future, my most heart-felt trust, and all the best qualities of the best that's in me!   I am doing this on behalf of myself and all my ancestors.

Feel free to have great expectations!

Our ancestors' experiences ripple down through the ages to us. Remember, we are the ancestors of our future. The healing we accomplish flows across time and space, and it can change everything.

Chapter 8:

Open The Cage of Overwhelm

Even though I get overwhelmed, but I swallow my real feelings, soldier on, and tough it out, I realize that is making me sick. I love and accept who I really am. I honor my deep inner strength, my truth and my goodness.

Here are two client stories about two very different sensitive people with very different lives. They both have resorted to numbing-out strategies to try to defend their vulnerability. The second story took place before I was using EFT, but it is a powerful example of how we think we must swallow what we feel and tough it out, and what happens when we touch the deeper truth of ourselves. And isn't that the message of "...I deeply and completely love and accept myself"?

Nicole is a sophomore in college. She came in with her usual bright smile, but soon it became apparent that she was suffering from feelings of overwhelm in all the important areas of her life, self-image, school, friends, relationships, family.

She told me that all her life she has been told that she "gets too upset." I have introduced her to the concept of the highly sensitive person. It helped her to know that there is not something wrong with her, though it is hard for her to remember that. She continually returns to the thought that there must be something wrong with her. She keeps apologizing for it.

Nicole starts out by saying she has been dieting, and she is so mad at herself about food. She is either eating or starving herself. Just this week she has had a realization - whenever a troubling thought or feeling comes up she reaches for something to eat to deflect her attention away from her discomfort.

I tell her how brilliant this is! So many people go through their entire lives medicating themselves in this way with food - or sex, or work, or drugs, or smoking – and they don't ever make the connection she just did. Nicole is bemused to be called brilliant when she is describing her terrible habits, but she takes it in.

There are so many issues that Nicole feels mired in, that we begin to work with EFT on just feeling overwhelmed in general, and she bursts into tears, sobbing for a moment, but also apologizing and trying to control herself because she does not usually express how she really feels to anyone (not even to herself), she just "toughs it out."

So we just tap up and down the points for a few minutes, and I come over to sit beside her to tap on her fingers while she cries and talks a bit. She is always amazed at how quickly and well EFT works.

Eventually, we work on her history of being told that she "gets too upset." I ask her how it feels in her body to be so sensitive – where does she feel that? She says she feels it in her chest, a warm heavy feeling resting on her chest.

(Often when people can't think of how to describe how something feels, I will ask questions like "Is it warmer or cooler? Is it heavier or lighter? Is it lighter or darker? Is there a color, or not? Is it a moving feeling or a still feeling?" People can almost always answer these questions.)

So we work with this feeling, and some specific incidents when she has felt it. I ask her to describe the feeling. Paradoxically, she says that even though the "too sensitive feeling" was warm and heavy on her chest, inside her it felt as if she were too light. And this feeling now of "getting too upset" is "heavier."

I talk a bit about the fact that many people overeat and gain weight because they unconsciously feel this sense of **too-lightness**, and want to add a sense of presence, even an intimidating presence. Consciously or unconsciously, they overeat to increase their "heaviness" in the world. Nicole is intrigued with this idea.

I also tell her about orthorexia, which is a kind of reverse of overeating. Orthorexia is an obsession with eating healthy food. It is related to anorexia, but is a different eating disorder. While an anorexic wants to lose weight, an orthorexic wants to feel pure, healthy and natural. (Learn more at http://orthorexia.com/) In a way, orthorexia is a rejection of the body, a wanting to be "lighter," even in a (distorted) spiritual sense.

I say "distorted" spiritual sense, because I believe that as human beings we are like distilled spiritual energy, literally "heavier" spirit. So when Nicole describes the too sensitive feeling as heavier, I hear her saying that she is experiencing her own spiritual Presence on the earth. A sense of **spiritual Presence** is an "inside job" of beliefs, self-image, perspectives and sense of purpose. Spiritual Presence is a sense of feeling full, full of one's Self, a *fulfilling*. There is a lot of creative languaging possible here.

I asked her to fill herself deeply with this sensation. Next I invited her to imagine having more of a sense of her spiritual Presence in those situations where in the past she had felt "too sensitive," as if there was something wrong with her.

We included all of this positive languaging in our rounds of tapping.

When we had finished, I asked Nicole to go inside again and check out her experience of those situations, now. When she opened her eyes she said, "Well, when I see it that way, there really isn't any problem!"

Nicole's experience reminds me of another session that I had many years ago with a man named Ron. I only saw him once, but his visit left a powerful image in my mind, and taught me much about sensitivity long before I heard the term, "highly sensitive person," and before I knew EFT.

Ron came in dressed in his work clothes. I had caught sight of him outside in his truck changing his t-shirt, and his jeans showed that he worked outside. It turned out that he did construction work. In his early 40's, rugged and weathered, he was not the kind of man who usually seeks out counseling help, so I knew he must be feeling desperate.

He had grown up in a loud, emotionally abusive, alcoholic family where there was a lot of criticism and little support. He'd had his own battles with alcohol, and with life itself. You could see it in his worn and lined face, his quiet sad demeanor. He was currently living in a situation where he was being unmercifully taken advantage of by his ex-wife, her teenage druggie son, AND her boyfriend, and he was supporting them all!

He thought he was being nice, and that this was what he was supposed to be doing… and he felt like he was drowning. He had no idea how to take control of his situation. He had no experience in understanding or verbalizing what he was feeling. He was truly overwhelmed.

Ron was so un-used to introspection that it took me awhile to find out how to ask him questions about himself that he could answer. I had asked him what he wanted in his life, and he had never been asked that before. He had never asked himself what he wanted. He didn't even know that it was possible to ask that question, and certainly didn't know what to say.

As a way in, I began by asking him to describe the worst things about the family he had grown up in and his situation now. That he could do. We made a long list. Then I went down the list item by item, and asked him to reverse each one. What is the opposite of a loud environment where everyone is yelling at each other? What is the opposite of constant criticism? What is the opposite of a situation where people are always drunk and unreliable, or violent? What is the opposite of living in a place where someone always has their hand out for a handout?

His responses were slow but thoughtful, and I could almost hear new neural pathways being formed as he tried to find feelings and images and then words for his new thoughts.

Ron and I worked through that list, and the result

it produced was a revelation to him. It touched my heart to see how sensitive he was under that tough laborer exterior. When he asked these questions of his heart, it knew the answers. That surprised him. I could see lights slowly going on inside.

Since I could see that he was such a different person than he appeared outwardly, or even knew himself, I asked him for some metaphors of what he was like "on the inside." He wasn't used to thinking symbolically, and he had mentioned a love of horses, so I asked him, "If you were a horse, what kind of horse would you be?"

And that is when his spirit started to speak.

Ron described a beautiful young filly, very high-strung, scared and nervous, backed into the corner of a paddock in a meadow. She felt trapped, tense, ready to flee at the slightest movement. She could not, would not be caught. Too terrified.

My heart in my mouth, maybe literally, I so, so gently asked him, using his experience and love of horses, did he know of a way to reach her, to touch her, to let her know that he meant her no harm.

He was kind of in an altered state as he talked, but he did not hesitate. He described moving very, very slowly, talking so softly, with such encouragement and love, taking all the time in the world to come to her. Slowly, slowly putting on her halter, and gently, quietly leading her to her stall.

And then, he said, he would slowly, slowly begin to pour corn into her stall, pouring and pouring until it came up over her feet… up around her legs… and up over her belly… talking softly and soothingly all the while… the grain slowly coming up to her withers…

and up to her back… and finally up around her neck.

I sat spellbound, listening as he talked, feeling something begin to quiet in him and come forward. I could feel this sensation emerging in myself as well.

And then, he said, when she felt the grain all around her she would feel held, and steadied, and *finally safe*. And that would change her.

A couple of weeks later, I got a phone call from Ron, canceling the next appointment we had made. He said he was quitting his job, selling his house and "moving out of the area." I took those developments as a good sign for him.

Even though there is no EFT in this story, I think that "feeling held, steadied and finally safe" is how we deserve to feel, and that EFT invites us to rest in this feeling inside.

Mapping the Cage of Overwhelm
Tough it Out

Here is how a map of the "Overwhelmed and Toughing it Out Cage" might look, based on real clients' stories. Now, co-creatively with the client, I can tap on each of these phrases, and weave them together to create new insights.

SENSITIVITY:

- I hate to be someone who needs special treatment
- It is overwhelming to think about being a canary in the coal mine

- I am too weak and crippled emotionally
- I am all alone and no one understands my pain
- I am sensitive, but I am not Mother Teresa
- I am too idealistic
- I am mediocre, an idealist who is not superb
- I am an artist who was forced to be an excellent mathematician and choose the sciences
- I would die rather than be seen as weak

PAINFUL EXPERIENCES FROM THE PAST (some titles)

- I Had the Wrong Dream
- She Said: "You Don't Have True Creativity"
- They Always Find Mistakes, Like Vultures
- My Father Said I Embarrassed Him
- Held Hostage at 12
- Totally Helpless

THE LIMITED IDENTITY I TOOK ON AS A RESULT

- I am defective
- It is going to be this way forever
- I have to do what they say for their approval
- My own thoughts and feelings don't count
- It is not OK to be the way I am
- I let everybody down
- I was shameful
- I will fail

- I am "difficult" if I don't do what they think is right
- "The only way to be solid is to be frozen"

RESPONSES - IN MY EMOTIONS

- Overwhelmed
- Anger
- Shame
- Deep sadness
- Discouraged
- Anguish
- Embarrassed
- Guilty
- Doomed

RESPONSES - IN MY BODY

- I grew up tough
- Can't feel what I feel
- Chronic Fatigue
- Heart is racing
- Want to cry but can't
- Heart feels constricted
- Constriction creeping up to my throat, closing off my tears
- Legs are shaking. They are saying "Get me out of here!"

POSITIVE INTENTION OF THE FEELINGS AND SYMPTOMS

- I was connecting to others' approval
- No one showed me how to approve of myself
- I am keeping my self in this awful situation to protect someone else
- I deserve to take care of myself instead!
- I can have my own dream!
- I deserve to open the cage my soul is trapped in
- "I **can** be in my favorite dress spinning and twirling in the wind and sunlight of the meadow"
- I can connect to myself

THE TRUTH ABOUT ME

- I am not the ugly duckling! I am a swan
- I am unique and gifted
- I don't have to lose my health to be who I really am
- I am good enough to be big and to shine
- I CAN BE ME, BE VISIBLE, AND BE HEARD
- I CAN BE **SELF**-ISH!

Feeling overwhelmed, and feeling like I have to tough it out, are signals to me.

They are not the problem. Those beliefs and feelings have created the problems.

I know how to take care of myself, and I intend to!

I deserve to honor my goodness.

Oh, my goodness!!!   :^)

Chapter 9:
Open The Cage of
"I Have to Be Perfect!"

Even though I live as if I am in a roomful of critics who cannot be made happy so that I always knock myself out to be perfect, I realize that I have been looking for approval in all the wrong places. I am learning to open to the strength INSIDE me. I choose to notice how I do things well!

Old Story, Scold Story.
New Story, True Story!

When I first began working with Don, he told me the litany of his woes, which were many. His life has definitely been challenging, and he now experiences many chronic physical ailments and debilitating emotional states of being. Don has spent the last 20 or so years seeking healing from every possible source, traditional to non-traditional. I remember thinking several times that he sounded very practiced at telling his own story.

We had had about four sessions. Each of them had been "successful." By the end of the session the issue we were working on had diminished in significance, and his physical and emotional symptoms were reduced and much less easily triggered. (I tested his responses repeatedly during and after the session.)

But the next time we talked, when I would ask Don how he was doing and how that issue was now, he would launch into the same old story about not wanting to change, it was too risky, the same problems showed up in his life, and he was feeling the same physical symptoms. However, I kept remembering that throughout these same sessions he had shared many interesting tales about adventures he had had in his life, the interesting things he was doing now and was looking forward to doing.

Two Different Stories

I got to thinking that Don had two very different stories going on in his head, and in his life, and he was only listening to one of them. I asked him to write me two paragraphs. One paragraph would be about the "old story," the very familiar sad one that he always told to his therapists and doctors and healer-types. The other paragraph would be a different story. I started out calling this the "new story," but I soon realized that really, it is the TRUE story.

It seemed to me that the "old" story must be in some mysterious way the one we were meant to live *through*, so that we could transform it by living it differently over time. The old story comes to us from our families, and from the emotional inheritance of our ancestors and our culture. It is about what seems possible for us in life. It shapes who and how we are in the world. And obligingly (it is a law of the universe after all), life shapes itself around us in response to what we think is true.

But - This Old Story Isn't WHO We Are!

The "new" TRUE story contains all the evidence of who we truly are, our deeper soul qualities, if you will, expressing through us in the activities and changes and opportunities we call into our lives. Even though, in the context of who we had been and were expected to be, these activities seemed surprising. Somehow they kept emerging from us in spite of ourselves.

I can think of so many things that I have done in my life that would not be expected of the child my parents thought they were raising. You probably can too, when you look at all that you have done in your life. I can see now, with the illumination of hindsight, that most of the terrible conflicts and sad times in my life were actually evidence of the Old and the True stories colliding.

Maybe I began life by unconsciously standing in my limiting beliefs about what was possible, in the emotional inheritance from my family and my ancestors and my culture. When the inner pressure of my True story got to be too much, I somehow burst through the limiting belief into an expression of a more natural truth for me—my real blueprint, as it were.

Over time, I have gotten used to my True story, and it would feel very confining and desperately uncomfortable to have to shrink back to the old one. I wouldn't want to. Perhaps I no longer have to burst flailing out of my limitations. It feels more like an emergence, an unfolding into what is really true for me.

I think that regular use of EFT helps to open the spaces between the bars of the cage of our limiting old stories, so that soon those spaces are big enough to step through, into a larger, truer story about us.

Another image comes to me: the "Chia pet" that has been advertised on American television. It looks like a small clay animal shape, with many small holes all over the body. When you water it, the seeds planted inside sprout and grow through the holes, forming a thick coat of lush growing green.

EFT waters the seeds planted inside us and helps our truth to grow!

Step off the Beaten Path

If we didn't have the pain, we might never notice the collision going on inside us between the sprouting seeds of our Truth and the limiting container of the old story that we are trying to live in. And so, with a tool like EFT, we can learn to BE our excellence. These are the paragraphs that Don wrote in response to my request:

THE OLD STORY

"The old story goes something like this: I find it very difficult to change. When I do change, or am looking at changing, it's always with a great deal of anguish and second-guessing, going over and over in my mind what the outcomes will be - they are mostly negative (as I see them). I view life from the perspective of the glass being half full and if something negative hasn't happened, just wait, it will!

"I strongly feel that I have a commitment phobia (really an addiction) in regard to relationships. I feel I also have a great deal of suppressed anger and when I get upset, rather than getting it out in constructive ways, I stuff it (I should not be angry, is a belief I have). I experience full body spasms, which are centered in my abdominal area and could very well be the bottled up anger and rage. I seem to be able to only feel the dense, heavy, negative emotions and very little of joy, love, and happiness.

"Change is to be looked at as something undesirable, for the most part, because I never know what is going to happen, so it's better to stay, most of the time, in my usual rut, even if it is quite uncomfortable. If I changed, things could get even worse, so I only change when it is absolutely necessary — and even then fight it all the way! While many people can seem to change with ease, change is very difficult, and in many cases impossible, for me."

THE NEW STORY

"The new story goes something like this:

"I have changed quite often and took many risks in my life. I've lived in many houses and apartments; owned many different cars; held many different jobs; went on trips to Europe, North Africa, Asia, Central and South

America, and Canada, as well as traveled to many different parts of the USA.

"I have changed my religious views and personal philosophy, leaving Catholicism behind in college (after beginning to question it in high school), later adopting Buddhism, and still later feeling more comfortable with a "spiritual" approach to life rather than being plugged into a formal religious structure. I have studied Zen Buddhism and Taoism; practiced and studied various meditation techniques, Tai Chi, Chi Kung, Aikido, and Kendo, learning something from each of them (I've studied with Shamans in Peru and from Russia; studied with Taoist and Tai Chi teachers in China and Taiwan; studied Kendo in Japan).

"I taught myself to fly fish and enjoyed many a day on beautiful rural trout streams. I went to massage school, after retiring from working 35 years in the employee benefit field, and began to develop a small massage and energetic healing practice. I sold my home several years ago and moved to another state after I met my love on a trip to China, and I overcame a severe allergy to cats in order to be with her (she has four cats). I also now have two cats! I received an MBA in my late 40's, going to school over a 3-year period to obtain the degree.

"I think I'm getting the point!!!!!!!!!!!!!!!!!!"

Write Your True Story

I invite and encourage YOU to write your old story, the one you are used to telling and hearing about yourself. And then look back over your life, select different events to highlight, and **re-write it as your True story**. Play with it a little. How would your life story read as a drama with you as the creative adventuresome hero/heroine? As a comedy, discovering yourself as the clever wise Kokopelli, the trickster symbol of happiness and joy? As a fairy-tale with you as the brave Prince or Princess? Or the King or Queen, for that matter. Or the Wizard or Priestess?

What we tell ourselves manifests itself in our lives.

Now create an EFT routine for yourself out of the collision of your Old Story and your True Story. Weave the two stories together into EFT set-up statements that feel right to you. Tap for them, and tap for whatever specific emotions and memories come up.

For instance, using Don's stories for some examples (you can find lots more):

- **Even though** I find it very difficult to change, *I accept myself and I accept who I am, and I choose to remember that I have changed quite often and I have taken many risks in my life.*

- **Even though** I have looked at changing with a great deal of anguish and second-guessing, going over and over in my mind what the outcomes will be, and they are mostly negative (as I see them), *I love and accept myself anyway, and I choose to remember and pay attention to all the times I have made changes and they turned out well, fascinating, fun and rewarding*.

• **Even though** I thought I had a commitment phobia, *I am choosing now to commit to myself, to expressing my Truth in my life, not someone else's expectations of me.*

• **Even though** my body spasms may be caged rage, and I have spent my life trying to heal them, *now when I accept who I really am inside, I can hear the message that my body is trying to send me: this is the collision of the old story I thought I had to live, and the True story growing inside me. I am choosing now to open the cage and free my spirit.*

• **Especially because** I have thought that change is very difficult, and in many cases impossible, for me, *I am glad that this apparent defect has gotten my attention, and I choose now to use it to open the way to Being my Excellence.*

Change the Shape of Your Life

It is absolutely possible to change the shape of your life by doing EFT. In my book, **The 8 Master Keys to Healing What Hurts**, I share the powerful healing story of Leila's life that threads its way throughout the book. Leila healed herself of 20 years of severe and debilitating fibromyalgia through diligent EFT tapping work and her persistent bright spirit. No one-minute wonder here! But her life now has taken quite a different shape.

The world responds to our thoughts and feelings, shaping life around us accordingly. Leila is still learning to maintain and continually open to this new shape, her True story, on a daily basis. You can see her at it in this email I got from her recently:

> "Next week I'll be making a trip down to my mother's to help her post surgery - knee replacement - age 82. I intend to make it a good trip, and hopefully she comes through the surgery OK.
>
> "In AlAnon I've finally come to the place in my 'growth' when it is time for me to make an amends to my mother for all the times I've hurt her - it's important that I genuinely do a 9th step with her - EVEN THOUGH she may not reciprocate with ANY admission of 'wrong-doing' on her part.
>
> "I must not expect anything - in fact, I must be prepared for just the opposite (more hurtful behavior from her towards me). This will take lots of courage and help from my higher power. It can't be a 'token' effort on my part.
>
> "So, when I get back, I'll be READY for your teleclass - that is for certain! (A ha! - just caught myself anticipating being in an 'upset' state when I get back - tut tut - talk about programming myself!)

"The truth is I'm just stumbling along here. I honestly want to have a loving connection with my mother. My life's lessons have shown me many times, that things will unfold in wonderful ways that I can't even imagine if I just let go and have faith - not fear. This must be true - I've seen it shown to me over an over - why not now with my most difficult relationship?

"I'M the one who has to let go of (and tap out) all of the old hurts - Time to tap on 'these old hurts', and 'this fear of my mother,' and to get even more specific with a few especially difficult memories. Then I won't feel at all anxious about finding the right moment to tell my mom how sorry I am for all the pain and worry I've caused her.

"Instead I will anticipate nothing but enjoyment from one end of the trip to the other - every day - no matter what. It's so beautiful on the coast at this time of the year - they get their springs so early. And I'll be seeing a couple of my children which will be wonderful - And I'll get a holiday from work here - And who knows what INCREDIBLE things will happen!

"This stuff is so amazing. Thank you so much Rue - your request to share my words has helped me to realize that if I spend a little more time on this before my trip, I can be so much more at ease with myself. Not just bravely facing the situation - but truly calm. "This whole process has been beyond anything I ever thought possible."

"I am changing how I define Perfection!"

Chapter 10:

Honoring Your Dark Angels

No matter what issues we are dealing with, learning to elicit the positive intention in a person or a situation is about the most powerful, heartening spiritual practice I can think of.

You probably have heard about "psychological reversals," or "emotional saboteurs." Maybe you know that the beginning set-up statement in EFT is designed to treat these reversals. I think of them as our internal goodness, distorted, that often seems to show up disguised as the problems in our lives.

At some point in our personal history, a particular behavior, symptom, or belief system appeared to be the best, or safest or maybe the only option available to us. It may still be operating in us now. It feels like who we are now, our identity. We don't question it. We soldier on with it. Maybe we got so used to doing/seeing/feeling that way that we didn't even notice when the saboteur began to cause more trouble than it solved.

But deep inside this behavior or thought or pain, there still glows the need and desire and *deserving of* the safety and fostering that we are still trying to get for ourselves. It is showing up distorted into a problem now, but there is goodness at its center.

A problem can be like a Dark Angel in our lives.

When EFT "doesn't work" it is often because we haven't yet identified the positive intention behind what seems to be the problem. When you are feeling under siege by an apparently negative emotion, behavior, symptom, or belief, ask the following questions - and expect interesting answers! Turn all the information you come up with into tapping set-up statements.

• What might be the positive intention of that emotion/behavior/symptom?
• If the part of you that is running that behavior were trying to get something for you, what would it be?
• This sure is getting my attention. What could be good about it?
• What is a context in which this would be useful behavior?
• If the part of me running this symptom/ behavior could have access to other, more powerful and much more effective strategies to get the safety/protection/love/attention it has been trying to get for me, would it be interested?

Hmmm...what else could I do to get what I really want? Should I keep the pain to make sure I learn the lesson?

I did a telephone session with a woman who asked a wonderful question relating to healing chronic pain. She has had fibromyalgia for 20 years. This was our first session, and she was just beginning to explore EFT as a treatment modality. She had done a little on her own, but hadn't worked with anyone else before using EFT in our session.

After I had gathered some information about her concerns, I asked what particular symptom or pain did she want to work with right now? Well, she said, she had a prior question she needed an answer to before we began.

Was there a chance, she asked, that EFT could be used as an "aversion strategy"? I asked her what she meant.

"I believe that life is meant to be experienced," she said, seriously. "I don't want to take away the pain if that means I am just taking the easy way out. Is there a lesson for me here that I will miss if EFT takes away the pain? I want to evolve! I don't want to foster the laziness in me. I don't want to not be proactive."

I found that very touching. Here she had been in pain for 20 years, and was willing to continue to be in pain if there was still something to be learned from it. Only someone really strong and determined could say that!

Or - someone who was "getting something" from enduring the pain.

How many of us believe that we must endure great hardship in order to evolve into our higher spiritual purpose? While I really honored her desire to learn and evolve, I thought her strength and willingness to "take it in the name of growth" were seriously misguided.

I personally don't believe that we are meant to suffer IN ORDER to learn. I do believe that our suffering is meant to get our attention, and let us know that there is something awry, something skewed in our personal belief system.

But I want to advance the heretical thought that we can learn just as easily, better, in fact, when we are relaxed and comfortable and looking forward to the creative possibilities instead of back toward all that we have not done perfectly. In my opinion, suffering seldom serves a higher purpose. I think that if it hurts, that is not good. I don't believe in "No pain, no gain!"

If this woman has been hurting for 20 years she is definitely not taking the easy way out! She is not lazy. But her strength and resolve are being misdirected. Positive intentions, bad strategy.

Soldiering On....
But Following Old Instructions

Coming back to that point about getting something from enduring the pain, it reminds me of a story that I heard about the Japanese soldiers in World War II.

In their book, **The Heart of the Mind**, Connirae and Steve Andreas tell about the Japanese garrisons of soldiers who remained on thousands of tiny islands in the Pacific Ocean. Most of these garrisons were dismantled after the war, but there had been so many that some were entirely missed.

The soldiers on these islands often took to the caves, struggling to stay alive and true to the mission that they took on to protect and defend their motherland. They maintained their tattered uniforms and rusting weapons as best they could, longing to be reunited with their central command. Even thirty years after the war had ended, these few remaining soldiers were still being encountered by natives, tourists, and/or fishing boats.

Consider the position of such a soldier.

As the Andreas' say:

"His government had called him, trained him, and sent him off to a jungle island to defend and protect his people against great external threat. As a loyal and obedient citizen, he had survived many privations and battles throughout the years of war. When the ebb and flow of battle passed him by, he was left alone or with a few other survivors. During all those years, he had carried on the battle in the best way he could, surviving against incredible odds. Despite the heat, the insects, and the jungle rains, he carried on, still loyal to the instructions given to him by his government so long ago."

They ask, "How should such a soldier be treated when he is found? It would be easy to ridicule him, or call him stupid to continue to fight a war that had been over for 30 years.

But the Japanese government, bless them, took a very different tack with these old soldiers.

The Andreas' continue:

"Instead, whenever one of these soldiers was located, the first contact was always made very carefully. Someone who had been a high ranking Japanese officer during the war would take his old uniform and samurai sword out of his closet, and

take an old military boat to the area where the lost soldier had been sighted.

"The officer would walk through the jungle, calling out for the soldier until he was found. When they met, the officer would thank the soldier, with tears in his eyes, for his loyalty and courage in continuing to defend his country for so many years. Then he would ask him about his experiences, and welcome him back.

"Only after some time would the soldier gently be told that the war was over, and that his country was at peace again, so that he would not have to fight any more. When he reached home he would be given a hero's welcome, with parades and medals, and crowds thanking him and celebrating his arduous struggle and his return and reunion with his people."

"I realized that parts of me are just like those soldiers"

I told this story once to a class of people learning EFT. As I finished, I noticed that one woman had tears spilling from her eyes. I asked her if she would be willing to talk about what she was experiencing. She said:

"I was feeling so sorry for those soldiers, and so moved by how they were treated, and then I realized that this is how I need to treat myself. For so long I have ridiculed or criticized or tried to shut away those parts of me that react so automatically in stuck ways that I don't like myself for.

"I could see how those parts of me are just like those soldiers. When I was little, the temper tantrum, or the crying might have worked, sort of, but those ways of dealing with hard times or difficult people don't work anymore. They just make things worse now! And then I just shut down, and grinned and bore it (but I wasn't doing much grinning). That doesn't work either.

"I have been still fighting battles that have long since ended, and then fighting with myself for doing that. But I can't seem to stop! I get so mad at myself! But hearing this story made me realize that there are parts of me that have just been trying to protect me and keep me safe, and they have been doing their best. But they just have those old tattered uniforms and rusty weapons that don't work any more.

"Some part of me is probably thinking, I have been this way for so long, I think of it as just who I am. And then the scary question comes – who would I be without these behaviors? How do I know who I really am?

"At least now I know that I should, and can, honor those old soldiers in me. They were just doing the best they could. They meant well. They were trying to protect me when I felt I couldn't protect myself. Once I honor them for what they were trying to get for me, maybe I can find other, better ways to get what I really want, deep inside."

What are your inner knights in shining armor?

Some of our common "inner soldiers" that have been working over time (and working overtime), have been trying to protect us from what we are afraid of. They might show up in our lives as pain, or illness, or allergies, or work-a-holism, or addictions, or anger, or overweight, or compulsions, or hyper-sensitivity, or...

These old soldiers may be trying to protect us from:

- responsibility
- new situations
- being seen
- failure
- success
- being overwhelmed
- being found out
- losing love
- being over-stimulated
- giving up guaranteed income
- getting a job
- becoming like our parents

When EFT "doesn't work," look to these examples of inner soldiers who are trying to help.

Tap for the resistance and the fear.

Here are some questions you can ask that might help to discover what YOUR Dark Angels are wanting for you. Use them in your EFT set up statements.

Ask inside:

- You, this part of me that is running this (anger, fear, overwhelm, pain, or...)_____, what are you trying to get for me?
- What are the benefits for me of feeling/ acting this way?
- *If I didn't have this _____ , what would I lose? What would be the downside?*

Use these questions to go deeper:

- So if I had _____(what I am trying to get), what would having that get for me that is even more important?

Or:

- When I have _____(what I am trying to get), how will having that benefit me?
- What becomes possible now?

If you keep asking these questions recursively, the answers will go deeper. Listen to your answers.

Maybe what I really want is attention, not healing. In fact, my unconscious mind might be thinking, if I actually healed, would I still get as much attention?

Maybe I am craving the surge of drama in my life that having the problem creates?

Maybe I am unconsciously thinking that if EFT works I won't have an excuse to: take care of myself / meditate / read / take self-help classes / take vacations /

or see all these practitioners of healing modalities.

Maybe the presenting issue is a red herring or smokescreen for the real issue(s). What is it keeping me from thinking about or feeling?

Maybe what I want is actually a "should", adopted to please someone else.

Maybe I've been working on anger, but it is really a cover for fear. (Or you've been working on fear, but it is a cover for grief. Or you have been working on sadness, but it is a cover for anger. Or...)

Be alert to the possibilities!

You can put the positive intention into the EFT set-up choice.

I have done a few here, just following my own intuition for the words. Try your hand at it. Doing this will help you to get a feel for the true, deeper intention that is getting distorted and showing up as the limiting behavior.

"Even though I don't want to get over this problem, and I am resisting getting over it with all my strength, I love and accept myself anyway, and I choose to find better ways of keeping myself safe."

"Even though I am too angry to get over this, I love and accept myself, I forgive myself for being angry, and I choose to learn how to stand up for myself in ways that feel better to me."

"Even though I will be too vulnerable if I get over this problem, I love and accept myself anyway, and I choose

to be surprised at how easy it is to discover my own inner strengths."

"Even though I might become powerful and successful if I heal this, and that really scares me because people who are powerful and successful are put down for being selfish - at least that's what my family believes, I love and accept myself anyway, and I choose to act powerfully and successfully in a way that includes other people and reflects their strengths. I can be humble and strong at the same time."

A Powerful Spiritual Practice

I always assume that if something is blocking the flow of spirit through a person toward manifesting the best of him or herself in the fullest possible way, that block has some positive intention. I think of it as a part of us that has been trying forever to get something for us, usually safety or protection. It is like a horse with blinders, a single-minded one-trick pony.

This part only knows how to do this one strategy, and it is stuck in the ON position. It doesn't realize that it is now causing you problems. It only notices that whatever it is so desperately trying to protect you from is getting worse, so it applies its strategy even more intensively.

I will ask, "Now, if this part of you could have access to other, more powerful and much more effective strategies to get the safety/protection/love/attention it has been trying to get for you, would it be interested?" The answer is always yes.

All of these questions make it possible to take the

basic, generic recipe of EFT, and design elegant phrasing that touches the hidden parts of our psyche, using the precise words that are the keys to freeing those parts that had been caged.

The "positive intention" questions and "Where do you feel that in your body?" are the two questions I ask most often, especially if some objection seems to be in the way of growth. I use them over and over, in every possible context. They are endlessly useful.

Here is another generative question to ask, when a person has begun to open to the flow of change within, and has a new sense of direction and choice. It is, "Tell me about a time in the past when you felt this positive way, or did this act of goodness." The purpose here is to reveal to the client that s/he has ALWAYS had this capacity to be smart, creative, loving, assertive, compassionate, even - *especially*, toward him/herself.

Maybe the whole cage that you have felt trapped in has had a positive intention. It has gotten your Attention.

It is a revelation to discover that
you have been good all along!

Chapter 11:
EFT for WOE is ME

Recently I slipped on the ice, fell hard, and broke my wrist.

I began tapping within seconds of falling. I lay on the path in shock and pain under the falling snow in the deserted park, all alone except for my two dogs who were milling helpfully around. Once I could tell that at least I hadn't broken a leg or a hip, and that my arm that wasn't holding the dog leash could move, I just tapped and tapped through the most basic points on my face and on top of my head. I was using the tip of the thumb of the glove on my only available hand, the hurting one.

I was in shock and not too coherent, so I didn't even bother with set-up phrases. I just repeated whatever words came to me, mostly what I was feeling, over and over as I tapped: "this pain,"" I fell," "in shock," "hurt my hand," "don't know if I can get up," "please help, (generic prayer)," "please help," this pain," "glad I didn't hit my head," "everything hurts," body in shock," "please help..."

I tapped like this until I was ready to try sitting up, and tapped some more until I was ready to try standing, and tapped some more as I tried to take little shuffling steps. I wasn't close to home, so I kept up this patter of saying the tapping phrases mentally, cradling with my hurting free hand at my chest, shuffling along gingerly through the snow restraining excited dogs.

Tapping became a kind of prayer

It was too much effort to do real or even mental tapping on the actual points. I assumed my body knew my intention. The phrases became a kind of prayer mixed with praise and encouragement for my body: "easy body," let this be easy," "steady body," "you are doing a good job," hand hurts," "scary to walk through the snowy slippery street," "you can do this," "one step at a time," "easy dogs," "slow, dogs," "everything hurts," "easy body," almost there," "slow and easy..."

Even in my shock, I was conscious of how important it was to avoid blaming myself, calling myself stupid, being angry at myself for slipping, or even for venturing out in the snow at all. I knew that how I talked to myself about this event would have major effects on my experience and my healing.

Even so. it didn't take long for my mind to go toward... "what a challenging year this has been for me personally... and now this...it's not fair...so much has happened already...it was already too much, overwhelming, and now this..." I began to incorporate those phrases and the tears that rose in me, first as I lay there after the fall, and then as I walked, and over the next days whenever I felt those feelings and thoughts come up. And they did.

Urgent Care tapping

I continued this tapping-praying-encouraging process on the way to Urgent Care (fortunately my husband was home and could drive me), in the waiting room, and even internally as the doctor manipulated my wrist and the X-ray tech took pictures from all the angles.

Getting the cast was another tapping opportunity. I could feel my body recoiling from it, feeling trapped and claustrophobic. (*Even though my body is feeling scared and claustrophobic and trapped by having a cast, I love and accept my body and I choose to allow this process to be easy and comfortable. I remember that this cast is to help me to heal and protect me from further hurt...*)

I also made regular use of EFT in the first few days to manage the pain, along with taking the homeopathic remedy Arnica, and the Bach Flower Essence Rescue Remedy. I had no need for painkillers after the first two nights of taking Ibuprofen to make sure I could sleep.

I am describing this experience at some length in the hope that you will remember to use tapping in the same way if you find yourself in an emergency situation. It is helpful to know that you don't always have to use the precise set-up structure. When your mind, body and emotions are in the grip of a powerful experience, that is enough. Tapping continuously, while you talk to yourself about what is happening and how you feel about it, can be extremely effective in the moment.

I want to say a little bit more about the effect of suffering on pain. By suffering I mean the story of worry and woe-is-me that we tell ourselves when bad things happen.

As the Buddhists say: "Pain is inevitable; suffering is optional."

Here are some words from Dr. Nancy Selfridge on pain and suffering. This is from the transcript of a presentation that she and I gave at the Association for Comprehensive Energy Psychology conference a few years ago:

The Difference Between Pain and Suffering

"When we're talking about a complex neurophysiologic process in the brain, we have to understand the difference between pain and suffering. Human beings across the board have a wide range of pain tolerance. You can shock one person, and they say, 'Eh, little buzz.' And another person, 'OW!' Right?

"The shock is not the difference. The difference is the experience of the shock. Now we have functional MRI studies that show that people who report a lot of pain have a lot of overactivity in the right prefrontal cortex, cingulate gyrus and amygdala. I call these the areas of suffering in the brain.

"People across the board with a painful stimulus will all have equal activity in the area of the brain that registers sensation and pain. That will look exactly alike on the MRI. But the people who report more pain, including your fibromyalgia and chronic pain patients, and those with a highly sensitive temperament, have hyperactivity in the suffering area of the brain. This is noteworthy.

"Dietrich Klinghardt is a well-known orthopedist and neuroscientist. He has talked in his literature about people who have gone through frontal lobe injuries who can report how much pain they're having and where it is, completely separate from a sense of suffering.

"You have to have an intact neo-cortex in order to experience suffering. When I tell that to my patients in pain, they say 'Can you just take away my neo-cortex?' I'll say to them, 'Oh, but we'd be taking a lot more brain function away than just the ability to think suffering thoughts!'"

Using Energy Therapy

So how do the interventions work when they do if we use energy therapy? I believe when we change our thought patterns we're going to see change in electrochemical flow in our brain from the limbic system. We can use some cognitive approaches but we also can manipulate subtle energies. I think these help to uncouple old established neurological patterns that are translated into pain.

Patients ask me, how does this work? I tell them it is sort of like running the defrag program on your computer. Whatever happened to you that triggered this real problem in your brain and over activated the suffering area in your brainÉthis area is sort of chaotic and fragmented with the information in there. When we do EFT it is like running a good defrag. That seems to be a model that probably is not very accurate, but it works.

Pain management = life story management = pain management

In other words, we are telling ourselves a constant mental and emotional story about what happened and what it means to us and what it means about us. This story can have an effect on how much pain we experience, and for how long.

So, using EFT to change the story can be life-changing! Literally!

Celia used to have a negative frame around everything

Listen to the wise words of Celia, who has spent the last two years dramatically re-writing her body's story about pain and suffering with EFT:

> **"Regarding 'REFRAMING'** - when I was ill, (fibromyalgia, chronic fatigue and post traumatic stress disorder) I found that my entire life's experience had a huge negative frame around it - and everything I thought fell into that frame in some fashion - even my more

'positive thoughts.'

"It wasn't until I started - very slowly at first - to learn how to put things into positive frames that I started to get better. So looking out the window - housebound - in so much pain - I used to think - "I'm SO sick - and I'm in SO much pain - and it's no WONDER - after all I've BEEN through!! "

"Then I started to learn how to look out the window - and see maybe a leaf or a cloud or even a twig !! And I would focus - really focus - on the beauty of what I was looking at, and I would think "Wow! I am SO lucky ! and SO grateful for all I've been through ! "

Focusing on the beauty instead of the pain

"The 'chemicals' produced in my body when I would coax myself to focus on the beauty instead of the pain - gradually - sometimes only for minutes - SHIFTED - until slowly, ever so slowly, it became easier and more automatic to stay in the positive for longer and longer .

"When I would slip - which was often at first - all I had to do was start tapping - (once I finally noticed that I was slipping !) :-) tap tap tap:

"'Even though I'm doing it AGAIN ! I'm STILL seeing things through muddy lenses !

"I DEEPLY and COMPLETELY love and accept myself anyway.... ,' *tapping around on negative thinking - (IF my resistance to the tapping would allow me to tap !) - which is a whole 'nother topic !*

"Also, at one point I put my 'addiction to negative thinking' and my 'addiction to fear' into the 12 steps and was blessed with more miracles.

"So now, these days, I have learned that if I allow myself to go back, to slip back into framing things negatively, the pain will start to come back.

"I get instant feedback for thinking gloomy thoughts!

"Talk about motivation !!"

Take good care of yourselves.

Give yourselves permission to eliminate or change ANYTHING in your power to change to make your life go more smoothly and easily.

Do your best to frame your days in beauty!

EFT can help.

111

Chapter 12:
Learn and Use EFT

What is EFT?

EFT is a rapid, highly effective, easy-to-learn self-healing technique.

Remember this, first and foremost:

All chronic pain - whether physical, emotional or mental - is about the story we tell ourselves about our experience.

I teach people an easy-to-learn method of dissolving anxiety and stress, easing both physical and emotional pain, releasing fears and negative or limiting beliefs of any kind. It is based on five thousand years of practical study in Chinese Medicine about the way the energy system of the body is affected by negative emotion.

This method works literally in a matter of minutes, replacing emotional distress with a form of peace, calm or confidence.

In essence EFT is like yoga for the emotions and the spirit, or a psychological version of acupuncture except that needles aren't necessary. EFT involves tapping gently on the stress relief points of the body with the fingertips, places we instinctively touch or rub anyway when we are upset, like around the eyes and on the chest.

Features:

- The results are usually long lasting.
- The process is relatively gentle.
- Most people can apply the techniques to themselves.
- It is inexpensive to learn and use, and easy to teach in a group while still maintaining individual privacy.
- It often provides relief for physical and emotional pain, headaches and addictive cravings.

Where it has been useful:

- EFT has been proven clinically effective in the Veterans Administration with many of our Vietnam War Veterans.
- It has helped in weight-loss programs and has also assisted students with "learning blocks."
- EFT has provided noticeable gains in many performance areas such as sports, music and public speaking. Those who meditate find that EFT allows them to "go deeper" and mental

health professionals are reporting dramatic improvements in their clients' well being.

For more information:

EFT does not do everything for everyone and is still in the experimental stage. However, the clinical results over the last 5 years have been remarkable. For more information, visit the EFT web site at: www.emofree.com

This is wonderful healing work that is easy to learn, highly effective, and an empowering self care tool that puts the ability to clear your path toward inner peace literally into your own hands. I think it is best to get started by working with an accomplished practitioner for a time to get experience and a sense of how to use these techniques creatively for greatest effectiveness. From there, you can heal your own life.

"EFT is astonishing both in its simplicity and its effectiveness in dislodging and removing emotional hurts and painful memories. I have found it powerful in healing present-time emotional pain (self hatred and self rejection) and in removing the hurt of events long past.

"I experienced liberation from difficult childhood experiences, and not only was the past healed, but I was empowered through the process so that my current habits of better self care were reinforced and strengthened."

(quote from a client)

The idea that, by using EFT, we can take greater responsibility for our own emotional and physical well-being is more than exciting.

The EFT Process:
(diagrams start on page 119)

The set-up statement:

A. Say statements 1 - 3 in a complete set three times as you strike the Karate Chop Point:

1. Even though I ____(insert your phrase here)____
2. I deeply and completely accept myself (or, if for a child: I'm a great kid, or another appropriate phrase)
3. and I choose _____(insert your phrase here)____

The Tapping Sequence:

B. Repeat the reminder phrase (the gist of the Even Though statement) as you tap on the face and body.

C. Repeat the reminder, or "I choose" phrase as you tap down the points on the face and body.

An example:

A. Striking the Karate Chop Point:

1. Even though I can't sleep
2. I deeply and completely accept myself
3. And I choose to sleep well and wake up refreshed.

B. Tapping the issue:

Repeat "can't sleep," "can't sleep," etc., as you tap on the points. Do two rounds minimum; do more if necessary.

C. Tapping the choice:

Repeat "sleep well," "awaken refreshed," "sleep well," "awaken refreshed," etc., as you tap on the points on the face and body.

Do a minimum of two rounds tapping; do more if it feels right. Add the Finger Points and/or The Gamut for stubborn issues.

On the following pages you will find illustrations of the various tapping points. Of these points, the most commonly referred to are the karate Chop point, the Sore Spots, and the Main Tapping Points. You will also see the Finger Points, the Gamut, and the Prosperity Procedure. Enjoy, and tap on everything.

Tapping Tips

The Karate Chop Point:

While it's OK to use the Karate Chop point of either hand, it's usually most convenient to tap the Karate Chop point of the non-dominant hand with the two fingertips of the dominant hand. For example, if you are right handed, you would tap the Karate Chop point on your left hand with the fingertips of your right hand.

Tapping intensity:

Tap solidly but never so hard as to hurt or bruise yourself.

Tapping and counting:

Tap about 7 times on each one of the tapping points. Because it might be difficult to count at the same time you repeat your phrases as you tap, if you are a little over or a little under 7 (5 to 9, for example) that will be usually be sufficient.

The points:

Each energy meridian has two end points. You need only tap on one end to balance out disruptions that may exist in it. These end points are near the surface of the body and are thus more readily accessed than other points along the energy meridians that may be more deeply buried.

117

Points on both sides of the body:

Most of the tapping points exist on either side of the body. It doesn't matter which side you use, nor does it matter if you switch sides during the sequence. For example, you can tap under your right eye and, later in the sequence, tap under your left arm.

Which hand?

It's OK to tap with either hand but most people prefer to use their dominant hand (i.e.: your right hand if you are right handed). Tap with the fingertips of your index finger and second finger. This covers a larger area than just tapping with one fingertip, and allows you to cover the tapping points more easily.

Excerpted from Gary Craig's EFT Course

Learn how to use EFT, and apply it to the many situations and symptoms of pain, fear, illness, anxiety you may have in your life. Use it to create a new and better life for yourself!

Go forth and prosper!

© *Rue Hass 2008*   *IntuitiveMentoring.com*
Profoundly light -hearted strategies for unsticking stuck stuff

THE KARATE CHOP POINT

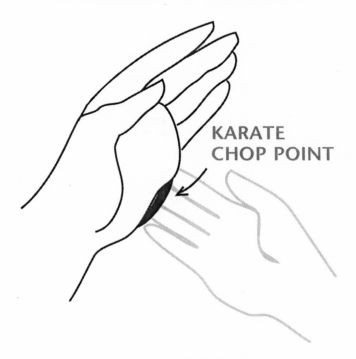

KARATE CHOP POINT

strike the Karate Chop Point gently with
either the tips of the first two fingers or
the inside of the combined flattened
fingers of the other hand

119

THE TAPPING SPOTS

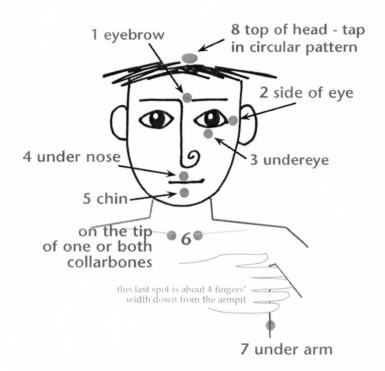

1 eyebrow

8 top of head - tap in circular pattern

2 side of eye

4 under nose

3 undereye

5 chin

on the tip of one or both collarbones 6

this last spot is about 4 fingers' width down from the armpit

7 under arm

THE FINGER POINTS

Use these points with the Gamut point to
pack more WOW into your session!

points are right
at the edge of
the fingernails

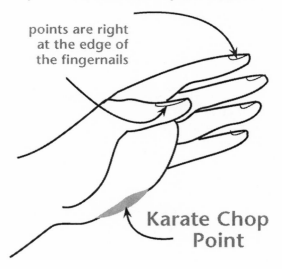

Karate Chop
Point

Starting at the side of the thumbnail nearest you,
then tap on the spot right next to the nail on
the edge of the fingernail on each finger
except the ring finger.

End up tapping on the Karate Chop point.

121

THE GAMUT

Add this step after tapping the face
& body, and/or Finger Points. It helps put the
body and brain back into balance.

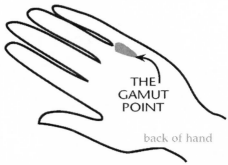

THE
GAMUT
POINT

back of hand

Rub the Gamut Spot (the V-shaped indentation on
the back of the hand at the base of the knuckles of
3rd and 4th fingers) as you go through these steps:

Looking straight forward (but relaxed!)
*and keeping your head **still**:*
1. Close the eyes
2. Open the eyes
3. Look down *(eyes move only!)* to the hard left
4. Look down *(eyes move only!)* to the hard right
5. Still without moving the head, do a wide rotation of
the eyes in one direction 360 degrees
6. Do a wide rotation of the eyes in the other
direction 360 degrees
7. Hum a few notes of a tune (like happy birthday to you)
8. Count from one to five
9. Hum a few notes of a tune

122

THE
TEMPORAL TAP
FOR PROSPERITY

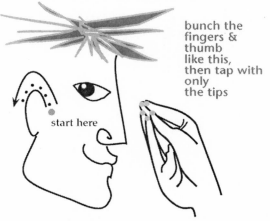

bunch the fingers & thumb like this, then tap with only the tips

start here

Bunch the tips of the thumb and fingers together
Start to tap where the right ear *(the right ear only!)*
leaves its connection to the face
Tap right next to the ear, but not on the ear
Do three rounds of: tapping up and around the ear,
ending halfway down the back down behind the ear
(as shown above), repeating this statement
(or a version you like better):

I graciously accept good, joy and prosperity into my life,
and all my needs are abundantly met, now and always.

Prosperity Phrasing by Michelle Hardwick

Chapter 13:
How Do I Know
What to Say with EFT?

My client, who has fibromyalgia, told me that the EFT work we did together in my office works really well for her, but when she gets home and tries to do EFT she can't figure out what to say. So we did a session on the pain she was feeling in her legs, and I tracked the questions I asked her and how we used her answers. Of course this doesn't cover everything possible to ask or say, but it might help guide someone else with the same puzzlements.

Ask yourself these questions, and any others that occur to you. Listen inside. Pay attention to thoughts, worries, images, physical sensations, feelings that arise. Tap for your answers! The phrases that we tapped for in this session are in italics.

- **Where specifically do you experience the pain?**

  Tops of my thighs, knees ("Even though I have pain in …")

- **What is the worst part?**

  My knees are weak, I can't trust them

(Even though my knees are weak... Even though I feel like I can't trust my knees...)

- **How would you describe it?**

  Soreness ("Even though I have soreness in...")

- **Like what?**

  Like an ache
  Knees ache ("Even though my knees ache...")
  Like my muscles are not toned ("Even though it feels like my muscles are not toned...")

(Continue to use each phrase in italics in this way, sometimes as a set up statement— "Even though...", and sometimes as phrases to say while tapping on each point)

(Note: there is no way to do this "wrong!" You can't do any harm, only good.)

- **When do you feel it? What triggers it?**

  When I am stressed and worried

- **When did it start?**

  Exhausted from exercise
  Tension in my body

- **When was the first time you felt something like this pain?**

  Some time after that auto accident ten years ago

(work with all the aspects of the incident)

- **Make a metaphor – what do your legs feel like?**

  As if they are waking up from hibernation,
  Like they haven't been used, no strength in them,
  like a bear coming out in spring

(I wove some imagery in later in the process: bears are powerful... feels so good to come out of that cave... the fierce protectiveness and will to survive and thrive of the mother bear for her cubs/you for your own body)

- **How do you feel about your legs hurting?**

It's embarrassing

- **What specifically is embarrassing?**

  I feel out of shape
  Walking that short distance should not be an issue
  Frustrated with my body
  Mad at my body

(Note: "What, specifically...? is an excellent question to ask to get deeper into vague answers. In EFT the more specific you can get, the better it works.)

- **If there were a deeper emotion under the pain, what would it be?**

  Worry that if I don't overcome this, pain in activity will get progressively worse
  Worry that the cycle of pain will get worse every time
  Worried what the future will be
  Anger — it's not fair!

- **What will that be like?**

  my physical abilities will be further limited
  physically I am not as strong as I want to be
  I think of myself as strong, but my body is keeping me back from that

- **When you worry how do you do that? (literally HOW)**

  a vicious mental circle:
  worry — exercise — pain — worry — stop exercise — worry ...a gerbil wheel of worry

(Pain almost gone... Here are some questions to ask to find new things to add after you say "Even though I have some remaining pain in my legs, I deeply and completely love and accept myself and…")

- **What do you want instead?**

  I want to fix my body, not mask the pain with drugs like my friend does
  I want a strong and healthy body

- **What state of being would you have to be in for this to be true?**

  excited about physical activity
  peace, health and well being
  knowing that I am enabling my body to feel good for my future

- **If you were no longer worrying, what would you do instead?**

  having new adventures, appreciating my body

- **I Choose:**

  to appreciate my health, my body

  ("Even though I only have a little pain left in my legs, I choose…")

- **What specifically do you want to appreciate about your health and your body?**

- **I Choose to appreciate:**

  my legs — that I can still walk
  my legs for holding me up all these years
  my legs for helping me to stand up for myself
  my arms, that they can give people hugs
  my body, that it can feel joy

- **I Choose:**

  to look forward to each new adventure
  to look forward to the future
  to put my attention toward what I want, not
  what I fear

Use your imagination, and your curiosity, and your associative thinking, and **especially** your humor to come up with images and phrases about the use and purpose, even the spiritual purpose, of "legs," in this case. Of course you can do this with any subject, and this is what makes EFT so fun, I think! Be as wild and dramatic in your imagination as you can. Let healing be joyful!

For example… legs support you, they are your greatest friends, legs allow you to stand tall, to stand up for yourself, to take a stand, to stand out, to take you places, to get you where you want to go, to take you away from what you want to avoid, jump for joy, run away, run to what you want, kick things out of the way, kick a path open for you, legs allow you to be flexible, be as short as you want or as tall as you are—in side and out…. etc. etc. etc.

*Now, sprinkle all these phrases in
as you tap along.*

Use your own imagination,
let it RUN free!

Give your intuition its own legs!

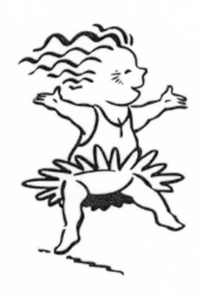

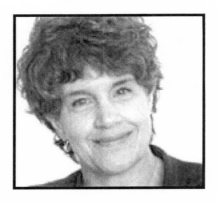

*Rue Anne Hass, M.A.,
EFT
MasterPractitioner*

Master EFT Practitioner, intuitive mentor/life path coach in Madison, Wisconsin since 1986 using *"profoundly lighthearted strategies for unsticking stuck stuff."*

I have been in private practice as an intuitive mentor/life path coach in Madison, Wisconsin since 1986 using what I think of as "profoundly lighthearted strategies for unsticking stuck stuff."

A long time ago, I was a college English teacher. From being a teacher I learned about how to learn, how to think about what was important, and how to communicate that clearly. I also learned that people in positions of authority are given respect whether they deserve it or not, and I set an intention for myself to deserve the respect I was given.

This was in the 1960's and early 70's, a time of a great creative ferment in the US and the world. I found myself in the center of this paradigm shift, deeply involved in the women's movement and the anti-war movement, living in an urban commune in Chicago that shared income, child care and household tasks. My job in our group was to take care of the household automobiles. (I was also teaching auto mechanics in a women's educational cooperative). From the experiences of this time I learned a sense of agency: that I had a place in the world, that we are all part of a bigger picture, that what I did and thought mattered.

For seven years, from 1974-1981, I was a staff member of the Findhorn Foundation, an international center for spiritual and holistic education in Scotland. Here, I was deeply challenged to learn and experience my own spiritual truth, independent of spiritual teachers and what other people said were the prerequisites for spiritual progress. I learned to surrender my prickly anger and the sense of personal "power over" in order to open to love and "power with".

Since then, I credit much of what I have learned in life to the bright enchantments and difficult challenges of motherhood and marriage.

My daughters are now in their 20's, beautiful young women from the inside out. I am profoundly honored that they set me up with their friends for counseling/ coaching sessions when I visit them. One is an acupuncturist in Denver, Colorado, and the other is in marketing in Boston, Massachusetts. I married Timothy at Findhorn. He works for an outpatient psychiatric unit, plays soccer, and would meditate all day if somebody paid him to. I think of him as a "mystic jock."

Over the years I have sought out extensive training in psycho-spiritual philosophy and therapies. Today, EFT is the centerpiece of my work. In January, 2006 I was honored to be named the 14th EFT Master. I love the simplicity and effectiveness of EFT, and the fact that it is a tool that people can take home with them. They don't always have to be going to the "expert" to get "fixed" because they are "broken." Now we have healing at our own fingertips!

What really powers me in my life is an intense curiosity about consciousness and a deep love of the world. I think of myself as a "Wise Woman in Training." (I have no intention of graduating! I will always be in training.)

In a first meeting with a new client/co-creative partner, I might walk them through an interesting process of understanding their life as a story, that I describe as "mapping the history of your future." It concludes with asking you to consider: "What do you want your life to leave in the world as a legacy. How do you want the world to be a better place for your having been here?"

I ask myself this question. What emerges for me is fostering in every way I can imagine, at all times, to my best ability, the concept of "Wealthbeing." This term popped into my head one day when I was thinking about the process of manifestation. To me, Wealthbeing means an interesting synthesis of "well-being" and "being (instead of having) wealth." I want to invite and assist people and communities to move into a sense of the real transformative power of their Wealthbeing, their own specific spiritual Presence in the world.